Sweet Surrender
Christian 12-Step Recovery from Food Addiction
By: Pam from Auburn, MA.

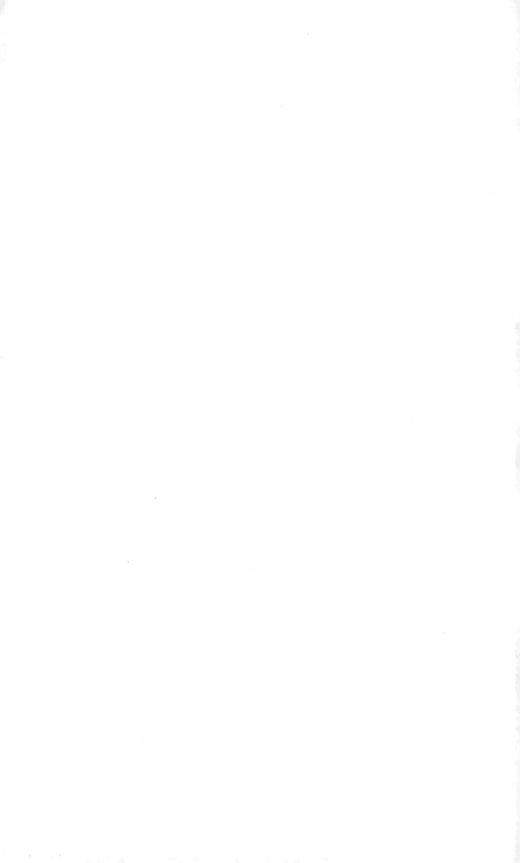

Sweet Surrender

Christian 12-Step recovery from food addiction

formerly Full of Faith (or full of food?): Christian 12-Step Recovery from Food Addiction

Copyright © 2004 by Pamela J. Masshardt

Includes Bibliographical references

It is with pleasure that I offer *Full of Faith (or full of food?)* to food addicts who wish to join me in recovery.

Table of Contents

DEDICATION

In loving memory of my mom, Lorraine, and to my dad, Donald Martin, my husband, Carl, my children, Dan and Joe and to overeaters and food addicts everywhere; God's grace and love to you forever.

ACKNOWLEDGEMENTS

To Jesus: Thank you for your never-ending goodness, mercy and grace.

To my son, Joe, my right-hand-man, technical advisor, prayer partner: This project would not have seen the light of day without your kind heart and incredible patience in teaching me basic computer skills, and your ability to design fulloffaith.com was a gift from the Lord. Thank you for your constant love, encouragement and assistance.

To my husband, Carl: Your love and support enabled me to accomplish what seemed like an impossible dream. Thank you for being my helper, financial advisor and my best friend.

To my son, Dan, and his wife, Heather: Thank you for your prayers and love from afar.

To my step-mom, Bev Martin: Your creative input helped me to move beyond the first chapter. Thank you.

To Allen Johnson, PhD, Lori Johnson, Charlie Douglas, RN, Gail Buckley and Nikki Gillotti: Your constructive criticism gave me knowledge, insight and understanding from unique perspectives. Thank you for believing in me. Your thoughtful words of encouragement kept me focused on my vision and purpose one page at a time.

To Pastor Douglas Geeze and the people at Faith Baptist Church in Auburn, MA: I will be forever grateful. You brought the Word of God to life for me (and my boys), and you taught us that Jesus (and the church) loves real people in the real world.

Introduction

Dare to Dream

Blessed are those who hunger and thirst for
righteousness, for they will be filled.

(Matthew 5:6, *New International Version*)

Over the Rainbow

Sitting on the edge of my seat, I nervously awaited my
cue to approach the podium. Pastor Doug was speaking on
addictions and all the things that separate us from God. I
was invited to share my story as a testimony of God's ability
to heal broken hearts, minds and bodies. "Lord, help me," I
prayed with nervous, yet hopeful and trusting anxiety. I
came from rags to riches. I was once a frightened woman
stuffed to the brink of explosion with food, lying on the
bathroom floor in despair. I had sobbed in desperation day

after day. Now I was, by God's amazing grace, qualified to speak about freedom and recovery. Who would have imagined?

Short moments seemed like interminable hours. I wondered what I would say. I prayed hard. Alone I could do nothing, but with God, all things were possible. "Please, Lord, speak through me. If it is Your will, use me to touch one heart, to help one hurting soul," I urgently cried out to God. The time had finally come. I took a long deep breath and walked up to the podium.

"Hi, I'm Pam, recovering food addict and co-dependent.* On July 23, 1988, I turned my will and my life over to the care of God as I understood Him. I said, 'Yes' to life and let go of a self-destructive habit that was killing me, physically, emotionally and spiritually. With the help of God, I stopped overeating one day at a time and God has been faithful to carry me from there." My words seemed to float into the sanctuary like precious bubbles. I saw compassionate nods and tear-streaked faces as the glistening of hope surrounded wounded hearts and spirits.

Over twenty years ago, God met me while on my knees. I didn't want to die, but didn't know how to live without food, my best friend. Among my half-eaten boxes and bags of food, I remained slumped in hopelessness day after day, week after week, month after month. I had seen a glimmer of hope in the 12-steps, but I was naturally defiant and strong-willed. It was years later when I finally admitted defeat.

*Co-dependent is the term used to describe a person who is recovering from unreasonable enmeshment in the lives of others.

The Cloud is Moving

Sweet Surrender is my story. It is my innermost thoughts and feelings as I trudged along the rough and rocky road toward recovery. Through the help of like-minded people, I learned how to live without excess food, and I found a God who was real and available. He touched my heart, soothed my restless spirit and continued to help me each new day.

Whether you are a full-blown food addict, like me, or are struggling with an uncomfortable feeling around a little extra food or a few extra pounds, we share common ground. From experience, I know what it feels like to be overweight, and I know what it feels like to finally hit a goal weight. Because of God's miracle-working power within me, I have maintained a seventy-five pound weight loss for over twenty years. Beyond physical health and a thin body, I have been blessed with peace of mind and a heartfelt desire to know God in a personal, life-changing way.

If my lifestyle appeals to you, *Sweet Surrender* offers recovery techniques and optional food plans. I invite you to join me in recovery as I share my story.

Reach for a Star

> "[Jesus said] ...even if you had faith as small as a mustard seed you   could say to this mountain, 'Move from here to there,' and it would move. Nothing would be impossible." (Matthew 17:20-21, *New Living Translation*)

Prayer changes things, and God can make what seems impossible, possible. He asked me to write this book in the year 2000. An ordinary woman, wife, mother and daycare provider with a high school education was asked *by God* to share the gifts that He had given to her. At first, I was flabbergasted with the thought of it, but I knew God was calling me to higher ground, so I said, "Okay, if You want me to do it, You'll get me through it."

At times of incredible struggle, disappointment and discouragement, I wanted to say, "This is too hard!", but I remembered that, "He who began a good work in me will be faithful to complete it."

Please, God, anoint these pages beyond mere words. Use this book, if it is Your will, to touch the hearts and homes of people who are thirsty for more; more God, more health, more peace.

Sweet Surrender exists to touch the hearts, minds, and souls of compulsive overeaters and food addicts everywhere with confident expectation of ongoing recovery through faith and hope in Jesus.

Chapter One

Realization—The Truth of the Matter

"I lie in the dust, completely discouraged..."

(Psalm 119:25, *New Living Translation*)

Perfect People and Other Myths

Growing up I had this wonderful fantasy. I would marry an athletic-looking man; we would live in a comfortable house with a beautiful, well-manicured lawn in a pleasant neighborhood. In the evening, I would be the perfect wife listening attentively to my husband and making pertinent comments as we discussed the events of his day. Soon we would be blessed with a child or two. I would be the perfect mother cooking nourishing meals and making sure my children were always happy. He would be the perfect father happily changing diapers when they were babies and playing sports with them when they were older. They would be clean, well-behaved and lovable. They would be perfect children. They would be one of our biggest delights. Every day our lives would be filled with bliss and happiness.

Unfortunately, somewhere on the road of life my fantasy took a wrong turn. I met Carl and we married. He was not the athletic-looking man of my fantasy world, but he was intelligent with a nice sense of humor. However, this intelligent man that I married had a terrible flaw. He was addicted to alcohol. When he started drinking, he could not stop. Unfortunately and unbeknownst to him, he also married a person with a terrible flaw. I was addicted to food. I was not a woman who overate occasionally, but a woman with a serious problem. Once I started eating, I could not stop. These addictions, along with some other instances of life's burdens, came frighteningly close to destroying our lives.

We did buy a house, a bona fide handy man special. It had no well-manicured lawn, but it was in a decent neighborhood, and it was ours. We did have children, two beautiful boys, Daniel and Joseph. They were my heart's delight. My whole world revolved around my children. I had succumbed to the idea that the perfect husband and the perfect house were unrealistic aspirations. Yet, I held tightly to the illusion of wonderful, well-mannered, perfect children. It was my earnest desire to be the perfect mother.

We plodded along reasonably well until 1980 when Carl lost his job after seventeen years of employment. It was not "personal." The company relocated to another part of the country. This was a time when business in America was suffering and new jobs were practically non-existent. Carl knocked on doors looking for employment while I sat at home worrying and stuffing myself with food.

Carl became a "jack of all trades." Installing rugs, working construction, delivering knives, he did whatever work he could find in hopes of gathering enough money to pay the ever-increasing pile of bills. Tending bar was his favorite. He met like-minded people and escaped from the concerns of the world. Many of these casual acquaintances helped him find lucrative leads to other moneymaking positions. We lived from paycheck to paycheck on the wings of a halfhearted prayer.

Occasionally my parents and my stepsister, Lorri, helped us by supplying food, shoes or clothing for the boys, but Carl was a proud man. He didn't take handouts easily. It was a tough place for me. Not knowing where to turn, I ate more food. At this time in our lives, fear and financial insecurity robbed us of any peace we may have had in our home.

One day my cousin, Linda, suggested we might help each other. Her infant daughter, Angela, needed a babysitter and I needed money. It was a welcomed solution. I helped Carl with our floundering finances while I continued to stay home with our children. Thus, my daycare career began. The news spread quickly. Soon I had a house full of children and a new goal: I would be the perfect parent/daycare provider to *all* the children in my care. It was yet another impossible dream. Just like my goals of a perfect husband, home and children, my estimation of excellence was more than unreasonable. My goals were unreachable by human standards. Therefore, anxiety and frustration consumed me. When my workday was over and my boys went to bed, I collapsed on the couch and ate junk food.

Early in life, I learned how to handle emotional turmoil. My mom would say, "Have a cookie, Pammy, that will make you feel better." It was like an old wives' tale, a myth for sure. I did not feel better after eating a cookie, a box of cookies or ten boxes of cookies. After eating the first few cookies, which was my usual intention, I lost sight of reason and my rampage would begin. Time after time, despite determined efforts to control my overeating, I gorged myself with food. With each bite, I sank lower into a pit of despondency. Whatever happened to my dreams of perfection? My hopes were lost in a deep sea of despair and a high mountain of food.

Cinderella Weighs in at 202 Pounds

One unforgettable morning, I crawled out of bed in my usual daze at the demands of my screaming year old son, Joe. On the way to the door, I caught a glimpse of my reflection in the mirror. It was not a pretty sight. I went back to the nightstand to grab my wire-rimmed eyeglasses to take a closer look. My too-small nightshirt clung tightly to my bellowing hips. My thighs jiggled like Jello and looked like cooked oatmeal. As I walked toward the mirror, I saw my long dark hair straggled around my puffy face. Tears welled in my eyes. What had happened to me?

My mother once told me a story about her best friend's mother. She was obese. Every time this mom came to school, the young girl cringed with embarrassment, almost mortified. The child often ignored her mother's presence and sometimes, worse than that, she denied that she knew her at all. *Ouch.* My heart fell to the floor with a loud thud. I saw that mother in MY mirror. *I refuse to be that mother. My diet starts today, no ifs, ands or buts. My children will never know that pain.*

I greeted Joe's wailing with a halfhearted smile. I was trying to be a "good" mom. As I rescued him from who-knows-what, his outlandish behavior stopped. Joe was just like me. He wanted what he wanted when he wanted it. The moment he opened his eyes, no matter what time it was, day or night, he expected to be released from the captivity of his crib, and he expected my full attention. I rarely slept because I refused to let him cry. God forbid, he might feel unloved or abandoned.

I scooped him up and headed back to my room to face the dreaded task of getting dressed. Rescuing my worn-out jeans from the pile of dirty laundry, I sucked in my gut to zipper them one more time. I couldn't face buying another size twenty. I dismissed the thought because today I was going to start my diet. I would soon be wearing smaller sizes. Determined to follow my food plan, I set forth to conquer my world. I kicked the laundry pile against the wall and thought about making the bed. *If anybody were to see this room, I'd die.* Joe and I went downstairs to the living room. I plunked him in front of the television set. *Thank you, God, for Sesame Street.*

Taking a moment to breathe and stretch, I felt the oh-too familiar wave of discouragement and groaned. My overeating was not my only problem. Our home was old and in sad repair. It wasn't the condition of the house that made me shudder, it was my irresponsibility with the cleaning—I didn't know how to clean, and I didn't care enough to learn or to do the work. My kitchen floor needed scrubbing, the living room needed vacuuming and the dust was piled high on the furniture. The laundry stayed in mounds here and there. Outdated magazines, papers and old mail covered the coffee table. Other things were tossed under the couches to give an appearance of a respectable dwelling. I didn't wash windows. It didn't even occur to me that people did seasonal cleaning. Basically, my house was run-down and unkempt, like me.

I looked at the clock and moaned again. My first daycare child was scheduled to arrive at 6:00 A.M. I have fifteen minutes to get myself breakfast before I begin my workday. Just then the door opened and in walked Jessica. Forcing a smile, I welcomed her, but inside I was angry. I wanted to eat my breakfast without worrying about more children. Obviously that didn't happen, but it was okay. Jessica happily joined Joe in the living room and I continue my mission.

I rummaged through my desk searching for my nutritionist's most recent suggestions. The sheets of paper were tattered and worn from the number of times I had played with them, the number of times I had attempted to follow the plan and the number of times I had thrown them in the air disgusted with my inability to succeed. This time was different. *Please, God, this time has to be different.*

Whenever I started a new diet, I felt obligated to update my weight chart. Hard as it was to see the consequences of my behavior, I went into the bathroom and removed every stitch of clothing before I stepped on the dreaded scale. I held my breath, as if that made a difference. I removed my eyeglasses and my rings. *Please, God, I pray that I didn't do too much damage this time.* Gathering my courage, I took the step. When I saw "two hundred and two," tears of unbelief welled in my eyes. I double-checked the reading. It was the same. *Yikes...I have gained ten pounds in two days. I am so sick. I need to stay on this diet today.*

I practically knew the food plan by heart. Breakfast was a serving of oatmeal, a cup of milk and a fruit. I quickly prepared and ate my breakfast. Other children were due to arrive at the daycare. Dan stumbled down the stairs, joined Joe and Jessica in front of the television and said, "I'm hungry. Mama, I want something to eat." Just like me, he thought it was time to eat as soon as his feet hit the floor. I gave him some graham crackers to share with his friends as they arrived.

Around 8 A.M. I grilled some English muffins to serve with breakfast. Dan ate the centers, but refused to eat the edges. Usually those were mine. I delighted in eating the leftovers. After all, my mother used to tell me that children were starving in Africa. It was my obligation to eat them. Somehow that made sense to me. *I am not going to eat the leftovers today. I don't need their food. I have a new diet. I can do this. I need to do this today.*

In daycare, meals and snacks are scheduled at regimented times. Snack time came quickly (10 A.M.). I tried to keep it simple by serving toast and juice, but the committee in my head started negotiating. *I could have a piece of toast if I eliminate the grain from lunch. I will be fine. Okay, I'll have one dry piece of toast.* One piece was not enough. The next piece had peanut butter and jelly on it. *I'll skip lunch. I WILL be fine.* In a heartbeat my somewhat composed disposition took a nosedive. Threads of anger bubbled within me. I started snapping at the children for no good reason. Distancing myself with a "don't look at me" sneer, I tried to overcome my fear of failure. *What is wrong with me? I can't even diet until lunch.*

Lunchtime was approaching and I wanted more food. Was I hungry? Who knows? *I already ate lunch at snack time. Please, God, help me. I can wait until dinner. I will barbeque a luscious T-bone steak, bake a potato and steam some vegetables. That is certainly a hearty meal. It will be wonderful.* Anticipation kept me focused for the rest of the afternoon.

I fed the children lunch. This time I threw the leftovers in the trash and smiled. *Wow, that was good.* I felt like a hero. *I can do this. I will be fine.* Later we baked corn muffins, and I made myself a cup of coffee instead of eating even one crumb. Patting myself on the back, I was pleased. *I am really good. I can do this.*

Dinnertime came. My mouth watered as I envisioned the delicious dinner I had planned. (It was like a love affair; I could not wait to be alone with my lover—the food.) In order to thoroughly enjoy my "date," I cooked dinner for the family first. Carl volunteered to entertain the boys while I cleaned up their dishes and ate my meal. I took advantage of the offer, served my bountiful feast on fine china, and sat at the head of the table all by myself. I felt like royalty. Eating one precious bite at a time, I spent nearly half an hour alone with my best friend, food. *This is great. I love this diet. I could do this forever.*

As I washed the rest of dishes, my mind raced to my next move, *oh no, my food is gone for the rest of the day. What am I going to do? I could watch television, but without food, it wouldn't be fun. I suppose I could review this new diet and plan my meals for the week. It would be better to think about the diet than to think about eating more food.*

Around 7 P.M. Dan and Joe were tired, and Carl's patience was wearing thin. In a matter of minutes, he was more than annoyed. It was my responsibility to protect the boys from his anger, but as usual, I joined him, yelling in an attempt to keep some semblance of a loving home life. What a tangled web, I yelled to keep him from yelling. Frustrated, I swished the boys off to bed.

It was my routine to read books and sing songs until the boys were asleep. So, as usual, I read their favorite stories and sang some soothing melodies, but this time my head was in the clouds; I was thinking about food. In time, the children settled down, and I joined my husband in the living room. *What can I do now?* Anxious and annoyed, I told my husband I wanted to catch up on some reading and suggested that he go to bed early. Carl was exhausted. He willingly agreed that he could use some extra sleep.

My pride kept me from telling Carl I was dieting again. I cannot count the times I thought I had the answer in some new and improved diet. It never changed anything. I would start off gung-ho only to fail once again. The embarrassment and shame was devastating. *This time will be different. I will prove that I can diet and succeed once and for all. I'll show him.*

Last Supper and Then Some

Everything looks different at night. The ghosts and the goblins come out of the woodwork, so to speak. That night all of my troubles were magnified. My burdens were too heavy to bear. My husband had problems, my children had problems, and I had problems. I wanted to fix everything and everybody. *Life should be easier.* I sat alone with no answers, no comfort and no food. I continued to dream. *Where is my fairy godmother?* I longed for a place, some fantasyland, where all the streets were paved with gold and everyone felt loved. Oh, what a glorious place that would be! Fairy tales are for princesses, not for me. I lived in the real world with real problems. Gloom and doom accompanied my somberness. *Poor Pammy, poor sad Pammy.*

Smothered by my insecurities and my fears, I remembered my mother's words, "Here, Pammy, have a cookie. That will make you feel better." *Maybe I could have a piece of fruit. The diet suggests two pieces a day, but three could surely be considered reasonable. Don't you think?* (The committee in my head concurred.) I scurried into the kitchen and found a beautiful apple. I grabbed my cutting board, my favorite paring knife and my special fork. Bringing my treasure to the living room, I artistically cut it into dinky, bite-sized pieces and slowly, carefully relished every mouthful. *That was okay. Apples are a healthy snack, only 60 or 70 calories. It takes 3,500 calories to gain a pound. I am still a "good" girl.*

Now what? I was hungry, or so I thought. I definitely wanted something more to eat. I pondered my options. It was only 8:40 P.M. The grocery stores were still open. *What should I do?* Marching to the kitchen, I began my hunt. Slowly and thoughtfully, I opened every cabinet door. My resolve to diet was waning. Fortunately, the cupboards were relatively empty. Food didn't last long in my house. I quickly ate whatever I bought. I felt relieved and considered going to bed, then a light bulb went off in my head. *Uh-oh, I'm in trouble now.*

Carl had some goodies put aside in his desk. I had promised not to touch them. He got rip-roaring mad when I ate his food. Once he even threatened to buy a lock and key to protect his stash. *I can't eat his stuff.* My history went before me. I ate his food time after time and then fabricated excuses for the missing sweets. Most often I pleaded, "Someone stopped by and I *needed* to offer them something." Sometimes I would say, "I gave the children your goodies as a special treat for exceptional behavior." I had to lie. The truth was unacceptable, even to me. At the time of the heist, I lost touch with reality. I was compelled. It was almost like an out-of-body experience.

Even though I knew it was wrong, once again I inspected Carl's hidden supply... chocolate kisses, peanut butter cups and chocolate covered cherries. *I could eat a peanut butter cup and replace it tomorrow. He won't even know.* Snatching my treat, as one might steal a kiss from a married man, I ventured back into the living room where I could fully enjoy this mouthwatering sensation. I slowly removed the wrapper. With anxious anticipation, I used my special knife to cut it into many tiny, bite-sized pieces. I slowly, lovingly devoured each morsel. *I love chocolate. I r-e-a-l-l-y love chocolate.* I was drawn back to Carl's hidden reserve and helped myself to the remaining splendor. *I'll start my new diet tomorrow. I didn't follow the plan today anyway. I had better go to the store and replace Carl's food.*

Gee, what else should I eat tonight? Chocolate chip ice cream, raw cookie dough and chocolate fudge frosting—maybe just a little of each. I could use some cookie dough to bake cookies with the daycare children tomorrow. It will be the craft project of the day and my excuse for shopping tonight.

Enthusiastically, I hopped in the car and headed to the market to buy replacements for Carl's candy. I also bought a bag of chocolate kisses for me, plus a half-gallon of ice cream, a stick of ready-made cookie dough and a can of fudge frosting. On the way to the checkout line, I grabbed a box of chocolate chip cookies for the boys. As I drove out of the parking lot, I rummaged through the bags searching for my beloved chocolate kisses. I downed six as I sped home, one mile down the road.

Gathering my bags from the car, I tiptoed into the house hoping everyone was still sleeping. I listened to the silence for a brief moment, but I was anxious for my tantalizing delights. I dashed to the kitchen and modestly scooped a reasonable portion of ice cream into my favorite bowl. I sliced four pieces from the stick of cookie dough and placed a dollop of frosting on each one. *I'm only going to have one bowl. I'll eat it slowly and r-e-a-l-l-y enjoy it. Normal people eat a bowl of ice cream and a few cookies as a snack. I have certainly had enough junk food today.*

Sitting in front of the television, I savored every bite. *That was so good. I want some more food. I guess it was stupid to think I could stop after one bowl. I am so sick. It has been less than two minutes and I need some more food.* Disgusted with my inability to control my eating, I hung my head in shame and retreated to the kitchen once again. I retrieved the half-gallon of ice cream from the freezer, the rest of the cookie dough and the wonderful chocolate frosting. I started eating directly from the containers, frantically concerned Carl might wander downstairs and notice my outrageous behavior once again. After all, my love affair with food was my precious secret.

Halfway through the frosting, I felt physically sick. My stomach felt as if it might explode. I got a bucket in case I threw up. *What is wrong with me? I don't want any more food, but I cannot stop eating.* I quickly dumped some filthy cigarette ashes into the partially eaten container of frosting, closed the lid and threw it in the trash. *Okay, good-bye frosting.* Somehow I ate the rest of the ice cream and polished off the cookie dough feeling a little worse with every bite.

Suddenly I had an idea. Maybe I should make myself throw up. Months earlier, a friend told me how to induce vomiting. She said it helped her to stay thin. I remembered her words. "Put a spoonful of mustard in a cup of water; drink it, dash for the bathroom." It sounded ridiculous until today. *If I can make myself throw up, I can eat and not get fat. That sounds pretty good to me.* I tried. God knows I tried, but it didn't happen. I tried shoving my finger down my throat. No luck. *I can't even throw up right. I am such a loser.* I gave up and started to cry. Moments later, I was face first on the bathroom floor sobbing uncontrollably. *What is wrong with me?*

My heart pumped wildly in my chest. *I am having a heart attack.* My stomach felt like a water balloon ready to burst. *I am going to die. I should wake up Carl and go to the hospital. No, I can't do that, if I have to tell him all I have eaten, he would think I was crazy. I am crazy.* I dragged myself into the living room and passed out on the couch until

Joey startled me with his crying once again. It was 5:30 A.M. I needed to get ready for a new day.

Back to the kitchen I went. My binge foods were gone. The boys' cookies were sitting on the counter. *I'll just have a couple.* I started with two. Two became four, then six, then eight. The whole row disappeared. Anger welled within me. I threw them on the floor, disgusted, and stomped them to death. As I discarded the cookie crumbs in the trash, I noticed the discarded can of frosting. I retrieved it, scraped off the ashes and ate the disgusting frosting. *I am really sick! Why can't I stop eating?*

I lost all control. Anything edible was mine. I concocted make-believe cookie dough: a little flour, some sugar, a blob of butter and a dash of vanilla. I mixed it all together and ate it. I found some old nuts, jimmies, chocolate chips and the like. Desperate and afraid, I sprayed oven cleaner on a batch of something. Convinced it was poison, I had a reprieve.

Minutes later, I found an old piecrust mix. I made pinwheels by spreading a little butter, a sprinkle of cinnamon and a spoonful of sugar on the dough. It took barely fifteen minutes to bake. As I waited, I found a stash of brownies in the freezer. I gnawed on one while the others defrosted in the microwave. I ate raw pudding mix moistened with a little hot water. I would continue to explain my rampage, but I blacked out here.

I cannot remember all I ate. It was volumes, enough to put on fifteen pounds in three days. I was sick and tired, but try as I might, I could not stop overeating. I didn't want to die, but I didn't know how to live. *Help me, Lord.*

Weighting in the Wilderness

"Ring-around-the-Rosy, a pocketful of posies. Ashes, ashes, we all fall down." I traveled around the same mountain doing the same things over and over again expecting different results. Diet after diet, I tried and failed. I could not stop overeating. My doctor sent me to a nutritionist. Her food plan was nutritionally sound. It looked great on paper, but it was the same mountain leading to another frenzy of compulsive overeating. I felt helpless, alone and afraid. The definition of frenzy in Webster's Dictionary explains it all: temporary insanity.

I was obsessed with being thin. I spent hours at the library seeking new approaches to losing weight. On the way home, I would stop at a store to pick up my last splurge. Any diet started with a binge. The Grapefruit Diet, The Cabbage

Soup Diet, The High Protein, Low Carbohydrate Diet, The Aids Diet Candy Regime, Atkins, The Slim Fast Diet, I tried them all. Nothing worked.

A special occasion, the high school reunion, the summer vacation or the holiday celebration always put me into a tailspin. To me, if you looked good, you were good. Fat was ugly and unacceptable. I would put my best foot forward and try, really try, to diet faithfully. With my eyes on the calendar, I often dropped a few pounds. However, as soon as the big day arrived, my usual eating regime returned followed by more compulsive overeating and more pain. My weight rose with each event.

Desperate for help, I considered weight loss programs. I invested in Weight Watchers, Diet Workshop, Gloria Stevens Fitness Center and others offered at local hospitals and medical centers. History repeated itself. I committed to a program, attended the meetings, and stepped on the scale (being careful to wear my lightest clothing). The next day was a free-for-all. For one day, I ate whatever I wanted. Then I would diet all week preparing for my next class, the weigh in and my reward of a day off. It was a vicious cycle.

Initially I experienced success, but soon rationalized and justified my need to stay home: "My husband and children need me, and we cannot afford to be spending money on frivolous things." Each time I stayed home, I made a solemn promise to continue to diet. Time after time, I tried. Time after time, I failed. Embarrassed, frustrated and confused, I could not understand why these techniques worked for so many people, but not for me. *What was wrong with me?*

Chapter Two

Acceptance—Real People in the Real World

"They will rebuild the ancient ruins and restore the places long devastated; they will renew the ruined cities that have been devastated for generations."

(Isaiah 61:4, *New International Version*)

Live and Learn

In the beginning was the word and the word was "food." It was not logical, fruitful or fulfilling, but it had passed from one generation to the next: "Food will make you feel better." Children learn to live from their parents, as they learned to live from their parents.

Have you ever heard "the ham story"? A mother and daughter are in the kitchen doing some preliminary preparations for a family celebration. As she had always done, the mom cut the ends off the ham and puts it in the oven. The daughter asks, "Mommy, why do you do that?"

She shrugs her shoulders and without much thought, she says, "Because that's what my mother does." The daughter goes into the living room where the other family members are mingling and addresses her grandmother. "Grandma, why do you cut the ends off a ham?" Her response comes without any question, "Because that's what my mother does." They turn to her mother, three generations down the line, for the answer. With a shy, almost embarrassed smile, the great grandmother says, "My roasting pan is rather small; I have to cut the ends off any ham weighing more than five-pounds in order to fit it into my pan."

Too often we don't question the why and wherefore of things. It is like using autopilot in an airplane. The pilot rests in the fact that the plane has been programmed properly. The question arises in our lives: What is the programming? What have we been taught through the years? When we open our eyes and see the truth, the whole truth, we have an opportunity to change. Cutting the cords to our self-destructive past performances, we grow confident in our

God-given abilities and strengths. People don't know what they don't know. We live and learn.

Goldilocks and Her Two Brothers

Throughout my childhood, my family was the typical mother, father, two boys and a girl scenario. As respected members of the community and the church, we lived in a nice little town in a quaint little house in New England. My mother was my hero. She was kind, caring, considerate and my best friend. Although she was not obese, my grandmother, all my aunts and most of my cousins were huge. Food was the answer to any problem in my family.

My twin brother, Ricky, resembled Mom with his small frame, light complexion, and blond curly hair. The family humorists say that when we were in my mother's womb, I must have squished poor little Ricky in the corner. "That's why he's so scrawny." Ricky was a sensitive child who struggled academically. I somehow felt it was my job to take care of him. I would often try to "feed him happy." Whenever food was served, I'd take mine and then ask for his. I was known to say, "Ricky will have a cookie." Little Ricky was not like me; it was a bother for him to eat meals, and snacks were a waste of time. I loved my little brother, but felt rejected when he said, "You eat it." Yet, I was happy to have more food. It was my consolation prize.

John, my older brother, was reasonably proportioned with light wiry hair and glasses. We had little in common. John was an intellectual. In my eyes, he lacked compassion. It hurt when he sang, "Tubby, Tubby two by four, couldn't get through the garden door." I was not exceptionally overweight as a child, but when he sang, I felt huge, unacceptable and unlovable.

Dad was a charmer and the love of my young life. He was tall, dark and handsome. At six feet, three inches and two hundred forty pounds, Dad towered over Mom. He seemed invincible, yet he was like a teddy bear, soft and cuddly. I was certainly Daddy's little girl.

As far back as I can remember Mom controlled our sweets by distributing allotted snacks. I politely ate my small, respectable bowl of ice cream or my one or two cookies with the family. Later, with no one in sight, I ignored the rules. Holding my spoon in one hand, the half-gallon of ice cream in the other, I ate. Be it a box of cookies or a pan of brownies, it didn't matter. I never intended to eat the whole bag or box of anything, but I was compelled. I could not stop. Panic and despair followed each episode. Constant battles warred in my head. To eat or not to eat, that was the question.

Halloween was a given, I ate. Pillowcase in hand, I was on a mission. When the porch lights went out, we hurried home to empty our bags on the living room floor. *I cannot eat my brothers' candy this year. If I got caught, I would be mortified* Mom told us to eat one piece a day. I tried. I really tried. My candy was gone in a day. Then I snuck into my brothers' bags and ate theirs. The love of food won over rational thinking every time. I kept looking for logic as I asked repeatedly, "What is wrong with me?"

I was fat, in my opinion, and I had two left feet. I hated being fat and clumsy, but I delighted in my family's reaction when I skinned my knee or bumped my head. My grandfather bought me candy and goodies every time I got hurt. Grandpa's rule was more pain, more gain. Once I tripped and fell on a piece of glass, cutting my elbow right to the bone. I waited anxiously for Grandpa's response. He gave me one dollar, a lousy dollar! I felt separated from Grandpa's love. To me, sugary treats looked like love, smelled like love and felt like love.

Family celebrations were wonderful. I happily volunteered to assist Mom anytime we entertained guests in our home. My delight was wrapped in thinking about, preparing and eating the food. I licked the spoons, cleaned the bowls with my fingers and sampled the results. My job, as a young teenager, was arranging the pastries on platters. All the imperfect pieces, or ones with the slightly burnt edges, were mine. I loved being behind the scenes, no small task for me. I had a plan and a goal: keep everyone happy, feed them, feed me.

By evening, I felt unacceptable, undesirable and unlovable. Therefore, cleanup was certainly better than talking with the people or hiding in a corner hoping to remain unnoticed. I took advantage of all the leftovers and ate off the guests' half-finished plates. I was stuffed to the brim dreading the next day when my new diet was to begin.

Humpty Dumpty Sat on a Wall

"Wake up, Pammy. It's time to get ready for church." I jumped out of bed and started rummaging through my closet. *What am I going to wear? I wish I were thin. I wish I hadn't eaten so much food yesterday, but it was a party. Everyone eats at parties. Please, God, help me stay on my diet today.*

Dressed in my brown hide-it-all skirt, I sat and listened to another sermon on God's love. *I wonder what the snack will be at coffee hour? God, help me to stay on my diet today.* Week after week, we sat in our family pew, the one invisibly marked with our name on it, listening to a similar message: if you follow the Ten Commandments and live a good life, all will be well. God was watching over his children. Heaven is a nice place where people go when they die. *When is the pastor going to say, "Amen"? I am getting hungry.* The usual greetings, the casual chitchat, and I was out the door investigating the food choices at coffee hour. I politely ate my two cookies. Not satisfied, I decided to rethink my plan. *Maybe two more and I'll skip my bread at lunch. I'll say, "I'm getting these cookies for Ricky."* Still wanting more, I grabbed a few and slid them into my purse for later. *Monday is a better day to start my diet anyway. Nobody starts a diet on Sunday. Today I'll eat. Tomorrow I'll diet.* People may have noticed my behavior. At first I cared, then it didn't matter. I needed more food.

Dad and John continually implied I would be happier if I were thin. I heard, "You have a pretty face. It's too bad you cannot control your weight." Lovingly John referred to me as pleasantly plump, which meant I was nice, but fat. Nearing my first year of high school, John became disgusted with my attempts to diet. He said, "You can't lose weight. Why bother? I'll give you twenty-five dollars if you lose twenty-five pounds." He had no intention of losing his precious twenty-five dollars. He was arrogant and insensitive. I was stubborn and headstrong. *I'll show you. Don't tell me I can't do it.* We were both amazed when I won the prize. I enjoyed a thin body for a few weeks or was it days?

I was a mystery to Mom and Dad. They tried to encourage me. I continued to fail. I appeared strong in public, but behind closed doors, I ate. I hid my boxes, bags and containers of food. Discouraged, embarrassed and humiliated I continued to cry, "What is wrong with me?"

Humpty Dumpty Had a Great Fall

Hope soared as I entered my junior year of high school. The peer pressure and my interest in boys created a positive mind-set. I was able to maintain a reasonable body weight for the first time in my life. I felt attractive. I found some friends, dated some respectable boys, and I participated in social events typical for my age. Then my world fell apart.

It was the summer of my senior year. Mom went into the hospital for a hysterectomy. The doctor said it was a common surgical procedure. There was no need to worry. Five or six days later, the bomb dropped. *What do you mean she's dead? You said it was a common, everyday operation. What am I going to do? Mom was my best friend. Why did she have to die? It's not fair. It's not fair. It's not fair.*

Alone in my room, I cried. Mom's words resounded in my head, "Have a cookie, Pammy, that will make you feel better." My self-esteem diminished. My self-control dropped out of sight. Alone and afraid I tried to hold the house together as chief cook and bottle washer. My dad and brothers tried their best to be supportive and encouraging, but it was tough. We all had our struggles to face.

My dieting dilemma returned with an added quest to find my perfect mate. After graduation from high school, I opted for a full-time job as a secretary at a well-known distribution center. My goal in life was to get married and have a lot of children. I envied my married friends who were starting families. They looked happy and content. They had a purpose. I needed a purpose.

I wandered through life searching for the answer to the question, "How can I get thin." *If I were thin, I would be happy. (Someone would love me. I would get married and have my babies.)* I spent my time at diet programs, exercise studios, health facilities, singles clubs, church socials, bars and shopping at the mall hoping to bump into someone special. But, no partner could be found. As the months sped by, I sunk lower and lower into a pit of despair.

Twinkle, Twinkle Little Star

Daily work was exceptionally boring with typing, dictation and filing. *I need something to eat.* It was around two o'clock in the afternoon. I pumped my handful of quarters into the candy machine and hit the button five times. I tucked the candy into my purse and proceeded to the ladies room. *I can't let anyone see me eating five candy bars. What would they think of me?* Hiding in one of the stalls, I quickly unwrapped and devoured all five in a matter of minutes hoping no one would interrupt my self-indulgent spree. Distraught with yet another episode of overeating, I went back to my desk and waited for the day to end. After work, I visited the mall hoping to gain a new perspective.

As I was walking into the front entrance, a fine-looking young man with beautiful brown eyes and light wavy hair approached me. He introduced himself and asked if he could talk to me for a minute. His name was Gary. My heart started beating. *Is this the one? Is this my perfect mate?*

It wasn't a minute into the conversation when I realized he was a "holy roller," a zealous spokesman for God. I told him I was fine; I went to church, or I used to go. I didn't drink. I never smoked. I never did drugs. I was a nice person.

He opened his tattered Bible and read some verses. Mesmerized I heard that everyone needs God. Everyone makes mistakes. God sent His only son, Jesus, to die an awful death on the cross to pay the price for our sins. He asked a simple question, "If you died tonight, are you sure you are going to heaven?" I thought for a minute and replied, "All people go to heaven, unless they are really bad, and God probably forgives them, too. God is a forgiving God." Gary looked at me in amazement. I nervously proclaimed, "I am a good girl." Defending my status, I started to blurt out some kind and loving things I did for people. He stopped me short and said, "You cannot earn your way to heaven."

I was getting annoyed. I spouted off in a brewing huff, "How do YOU know you are going to heaven?" He didn't react to my brash attitude. His calm demeanor stayed firm as he explained his position. "I acknowledged my need for God, admitted I was a sinner and asked for God to forgive me. I know from the Word of God, The Bible, Jesus died for my sins. I invited Him into my heart. He is my Lord and Savior."

Gary showed me some verses in the Bible: God's Purpose: Romans 5:1, John 3:16, Our Problem: Romans 3:23, 6:23, Our Powerlessness: Proverbs 14:12, Isaiah 59:2, The Solution: 1 Timothy 2:5, 1 Peter 3:18a, Romans 5:8, Our Choice: Revelations 3:20, John 1:12, Romans 10:9, Assurance: Romans 10:13, Ephesians 2:8-9.

After some heartfelt twinges, I asked him what I needed to do to get right with God. He said it was simple. "If you believe what I have told you, tell God how you feel." I sat and pondered my choices. In a few brief moments, I knew what I needed to do. Timidly I welcomed Jesus into my heart and my life.

"God, I have made lots of mistakes in my life. I am sorry. The Bible tells me that everyone makes mistakes; it is the human condition. No matter how hard I try, I cannot be perfect. That's why I need you, Lord Jesus. Please help me to know and do Your will today. I thought that everyone went to heaven when they died. I now see Your message of hope is for believers. I believe that the Bible is The Word of God. I believe that You died so that I could live. Your Holy Spirit will guide me and help me in this life, and I will see You face-to-face one day in the next. Thank You, Lord, for this amazing gift. Amen."

Thirsty for more information about God, I went to the religious bookstore with eager anticipation and purchased a beautiful, leather-bound Bible. A woman in the store suggested the King James Version. I had my name boldly imprinted on the cover. I knew my life would never be the same again.

Alone in my room, I opened my precious new Bible. I started reading...*Adam and Eve, Cain, Abel and Seth—what do they have to do with my life?* I glanced ahead, flipped through some pages. It was like a foreign language to me. Confused and disappointed, I put the Bible on my bedside table and continued my search for the perfect diet and the perfect mate.

Jack and Jill Went Up the Hill

Years went by. Dad married one of the secretaries where he worked. John married a girl he met in college. Ricky married a girl from the lake where we had our summer home. Still alone, I sat in my apartment and wept. *"What is wrong with me?"*

Thank God for my job. Five years as the secretary to the purchasing agent at a large well-known distribution center proved I had some worth and value. I loved my job and I did it well.

"Pam, did you hear about the new job?" The word spread quickly; a new position was created in the warehouse of two hundred fifty men and a few women. *If you want a man, go where the men are.* It was a division of the Personnel Department, a one-girl office. I was overly qualified, but the company agreed to move me laterally. I wanted that job.

I had constant contact with men. I was the woman to see for any personnel problems or concerns. My title was Administrative Assistant, which meant receptionist, payroll clerk, insurance claims coordinator and secretary to the warehouse manager. It was the perfect job for me.

Carl was the working supervisor of the Parcel Post Department. "Hi, Carl, how's it going today?" I said. He was friendly, but not my type. He was small, kind of gruff-looking and divorced with four children. We found common ground by the copy machine. I had problems. He had problems. In time, we became dependent on each other. It only made sense that we should marry, so we did.

Carl knew my heart. We had talked about children for hours before we were married. I would be an at-home mom. He liked being a dad. Due to complicated circumstances, it was difficult to fulfill his role as a father to his four girls, and I was too self-centered to understand my responsibilities as stepmother. Daniel was born in 1980. Being Mom was not as I had expected. Nothing ever was. It was hard work. We had serious problems. Carl drank and I ate. Daniel needed a playmate. Joseph was born in 1983.

My parenting skills were as I had been taught from my own experiences. "Here, Danny, have a cookie. That will make you feel better." It was the "don't feel" answer to any problem. I taught my boys well. They were invited to my eating frenzies, respectably called a party. We planned a celebration for one reason or another and bought the appropriate party supplies, lots of food. Still intending to enjoy only one piece or bowl, we began the festivities. It was fun for the first five minutes. The boys ate their treats and wandered off to play, leaving me alone with the food. One slice of cake was never enough. I slivered a little from one side, slivered a little from the other; eventually I devoured the whole thing or the familiar regime with ice cream, one spoonful led to two, to three, to consuming the whole container. I was sick and tired of being sick and tired, but I could not stop overeating. I tried. God knows I tried day after day. My overeating splurges evolved into a way of life, coupled with frustration, hurt, disappointment and rage.

My poor children, God bless them. They had a loving mother one minute, when my diet was going well or a screaming maniac the next, when my diet was abandoned one more time. I was physically and emotionally exhausted, hopeless and full of despair.

My binges were more often and more severe. Raw chocolate chip cookie dough, chocolate fudge frosting and a half-gallon of ice cream, that's where I began. Anything edible followed. I ate until the food was gone or I passed out, whichever came first.

Desperate and fearful for my health and life, alone in the confines of my mind, I begged God to show me a way out of my misery. *Help me, Lord. I do not want to die and abandon my children. There has to be more to life than this. I am begging you, Lord. Help me, please.*

I didn't know many verses in the Bible, but I remembered Mom wearing a necklace with a mustard seed pendent. She told me the story about faith. She said, "If you have faith as small as a mustard seed, God can help you."

"...Anything is possible if you have faith... I *do* have faith; oh, help me to have *more!"* (Mark 9:23-24, *The Living Bible*)

Jack Fell Down

I felt like a single parent, fully responsible for the children and our home. Carl worked most days and nights. One day he came home all excited. His words gushed like a babbling brook, "Baby [we always called each other "baby"] Baby, I got a job. It's our dream-come-true. I'll be working at the utility company. For six months it will be tough, but after that we'll be fine." *Yahoo, we are finally on our way to happiness. Thank you, God.* We rejoiced and were glad.

The months rolled by. Nothing changed. He still worked many hours, came home and passed out on the couch. His new job was flexible. He could have come home after work, sometimes as early as 11:30 A.M., but he never wanted to be with the "bunches of children hanging on the furniture." That's how he described the daycare.

"Dad, can the boys and I come stay with you for a few days? I am leaving Carl." Sad as the situation was, my father welcomed us with open arms. *I love my daddy. I am still his little girl.*

Outside of close family members (Dad, my stepmother and my stepsister, Lorri), no one knew I was troubled, not even Carl. I had been taught to keep secrets. My mother would say, "We don't talk about our problems; we don't show the neighbors our dirty laundry." Simplified, "Shut up. Keep the peace at all cost."

Carl went fishing. He came home to a note on the table. "We're at Dad's. I won't be back." Shocked and dismayed, he was breathless. I blamed all our problems on him and his drinking. I thought that if he were sober, we would have that storybook family life like Ozzie and Harriet, and I wouldn't overeat. I would be fine, if he would just stop drinking.

Carl asked if I would help him get sober. He said, "Baby, come home for three months. If I take even one drink, you can leave." I loved him. I hated the alcohol. It was a fair deal.

And Broke His Crown

A banner hung from the blackboard, "The Twelve Steps." My eyes were drawn to the words, "Came to believe that a power greater than ourselves could restore us to sanity." *Sanity...what's that?*

With apprehension and fear, we attended a recovery group for alcoholics. I went to support and encourage Carl's newfound hope of sobriety. We found some seats in the dreary, smoke-filled room. I glanced around at our counterparts. It was certainly a mixed bag of people, mostly regular folk like us.

Men and women shared bits and pieces of their lives, the good, bad and the ugly. I heard some amazing things that first night. "Alcoholism is a debilitating sickness. It is progressive and can be fatal. It affects the whole family." I cried and I laughed. Somewhat baffled, I knew these people were talking directly to ME. I marveled at their honesty. *These people are showing me their "dirty laundry." They have secrets like me. I am not unique. Carl is not the only addict in this family.*

One woman was talking about having "just one glass" of wine with a meal. "After all, it was a celebration." She could not stop. I could relate. One piece of birthday cake or one cookie, stopping never happened for me either.

The man dressed in black was discouraged. I nodded in agreement when he said, "What is wrong with me?" He tried to do controlled drinking. "I'll only drink beer and no hard stuff," "I'll only drink after 8 P.M.," "I'll dilute the alcohol in milk." He failed every time.

"When a normal person discovers that he has a flat tire, he calls the garage. When an alcoholic gets a flat, he calls suicide prevention." *Yup, that's me, too, extreme in everything*. A calm sense of peace came over me. I felt hopeful. Carl was sober. Maybe I could win over my addiction, too. "It is just one day at a time." *Tomorrow I'll begin my diet*. The meeting ended with the Serenity Prayer.

And Jill Came Tumbling After

A good-intentioned friend visited us and gave Carl a book that he referred to as "The Big Book." He said that he was an alcoholic and this was the "Bible" of the program that worked for him. I grabbed it before Carl could say a word and said, "Can I read it? I *know* that I am an addict. Sweets are my alcohol." Our friend released it to me with a smile. However, Carl looked at me as if I were crazy. He rolled his eyes and said sternly, "Food is not like alcohol." Under my breath I mumbled, "I'll show you." I was serious and confident God had given me my answer.

As soon as I was alone, I read Bill's story. He was the founding father of Alcoholics Anonymous, an interesting man, mixed-up and unbalanced like me. I recognized my warped, exaggerated imagination, my lost reasoning and my lack of self-control. *I am an addict. Addiction is addiction. I know God wants me to be happy and healthy. Diets don't work. Okay, God, help me to apply these principles to my food problem.* "The Twelve Steps are the map of the program," echoed in my mind.

Step one: We admitted we were powerless over food, that our lives had become unmanageable. *No doubt. I think about food day and night. I try to control myself, but I cannot stop overeating even though I know bingeing and starving is harmful and possibly fatal. I don't want to die, but I don't know how to live.*

I pondered **Step two: Came to believe that a power greater than ourselves could restore us to sanity.** According to Webster's Dictionary, sanity is freedom from mental derangement, being reasonable and sensible. *I need sanity in my life.* A memory of my mother flashed before me. She was teaching me lullabies one restless night. "Jesus loves me this I know for the Bible tells me so." *I believe in a power greater than myself. I believe in God. Yes, most assuredly. I will never forget my experience in the mall years ago, and I know God brought me to Alcoholics Anonymous to teach me how to live without sugar. I will learn to live as a recovering addict.*

Step three: Made the decision to turn our will and our lives over to the care of God, *as we understood him. Okay, God, I believe you want me to be free from my addiction. I will stop eating my "alcohol." I will stop eating sugar-laden junk food.* The program emphasizes one day at a time. I made the decision: no sugar for one day.

My day began with a healthy breakfast: a grilled bagel, an egg and a banana with my pot of coffee. I felt fine for about ten minutes. Then my head started to spin. By noon, I was eating anything and everything once again. *I am not an alcoholic. Food is different, not like alcohol or drugs. People who drink excessively act inappropriately, trip and stumble, slur their words, pass out on park benches. No one even knows I have a problem. Besides, how bad can it be? Every church has sweets and treats mingled into celebrations, meetings and social affairs. People are asked to enjoy the food. To apply the steps of Alcoholics Anonymous to my problem is foolish thinking. Carl is right. I am crazy. I was grasping at straws and employing desperate thinking. Food is not like alcohol. There must be another answer for me.*

Chapter Three

Surrender—Addiction is Real, Debilitating and Ultimately fatal

"He lifted me out of the pit of despair, out of the mud and the mire. He set my feet on solid ground and steadied me as I walked along."

(Psalm 40:2, *New Living Translation*)

Sparks of Light

Carl was recovering one day at a time. It was a miracle. He learned how to live without alcohol. I watched him with amazement as I continued my search. The days and months rolled by. Hopeless and helpless, I was as desperate as the dying can be.

In lieu of eating yet another bite of whatever, I grabbed the Sunday newspaper and scanned the classified section for feasible options. A 12-step program caught my eye. Nervously I dialed the number. The phone rang what seemed like fifteen hundred times. Finally, a soft-spoken woman answered. I asked if she would send me the diet. I explained that meetings might not work for me. It was hard getting out of the house, leaving the kids and all. I remember her gentle chuckle as she replied, "This program does not promote any food plans." She graciously offered to send me some information. Two days later, my newcomer packet arrived, along with a questionnaire. My very first inventory looked something like this. (*15 Questions*, Copyright l986. Reprinted by permission from the publisher).

1. Do you eat when you're not hungry?

Yes, I eat for other reasons, including anxiety, frustration, boredom and the like.

2. Do you go on eating binges for no apparent reason?

Some of my binges are not planned. Most of my binges are not planned. I make a decision to have a small, reasonable portion (two cookies or a candy bar) My one or two pieces become four, then six, then eight until the whole bag or box disappears. I know in my head I need to stop. I want to stop, but I continue to raid the cabinets searching for more food. Feeling like a failure, I think, "I might as well continue to eat today. Tomorrow I will start my diet." I pray for the ability to stop as I consume whatever I can find, the better quality foods first. Then whatever appeases my appetite for the moment. Nothing satisfies my hunger. I go into a trance. I have absolutely no control.

3. Do you have feelings of guilt and remorse after overeating?

I feel like a failure. I should be able to control my eating. Why can't I stop eating? It makes no sense to me.

4. Do you give too much time and thought to food?

I think of food all the time. I am forever trying to control my diet. Plus, it seems all our fun times are planned around food. For me, special foods are associated with different events—ice cream, fried dough and fudge at the beach or S'mores and popcorn by the fire at a campground or hot chocolate with marshmallows and doughnuts at a winter outing.

5. Do you look forward with pleasure and anticipation to the time when you can eat alone?

I love to eat alone. When my husband has to work late or has an evening meeting to attend, I set up my plan for the night. I wait until the boys are in bed and begin my rendezvous with the food: an elaborate dinner and an extraordinary dessert. More times than not, it leads into an explosive free-for-all binge.

6. Do you plan these secret binges ahead of time?

Whenever I find a new diet, I need a day to prepare. I eat all the things that I will "never have again." I also give myself permission to enjoy special days or a holiday season or wonderful vacations.

7. Do you eat sensibly before others and make up for it alone?

I can make a good impression by eating reasonable portions in front of people. It is embarrassing to be overweight and overeating. In a stressful situation or even a celebration, my mind is rushing to the reward coming. Alone I can enjoy my food.

8. Is your weight affecting the way you live your life?

Dad refers to me as "happy go lucky." The truth is I am not happy. Most assuredly my weight is affecting my life. I should not feel so distraught. I have a nice home, a husband who loves and supports the family and two wonderful children whom I adore.

Carl and I have had our difficulties, but we are okay. I know it is God's will for me to be a responsible, loving parent and a caring wife. I am successful most of the time; however, I could be kind and loving one minute, when I am in control of my food and having a "good" day on my diet, and then on a "bad" day, I am like another person—some eccentric lunatic. My poor husband and children are ignored or worse, I get angry. I start banging cabinet doors and complaining about everything and everybody.

By the grace of God, I have the ability to save most of my overeating until late evenings. Then I can refrain from hurting the people I love. I am alone with my food. The only victim for my abusive thoughts and actions is myself. Outside the home, when I am obliged to attend a social affair or a sporting event, I sit somewhere hoping to remain unnoticed. I am ashamed of my size and my lack of grace. I waddle when I walk. I fear people judging me, as I am judging them—fat is ugly. Thin is beautiful. I would prefer staying home where I am safe and secure in my private little world.

9. Have you tried to diet for a week (or longer), only to fall short of your goals?

I have been successful at times for a week or more, but never long-term. I give up and go back to my normal eating habits. Maybe I need to accept myself as a fat person. Some people say I am big boned. I see overweight women on television who are happy. They say, "Big is beautiful." I don't agree. Thin is beautiful. It is my hope, my dream and my vision to be thin.

10. Do you resent others telling you to "use a little willpower" to stop overeating?

I want to yell and scream, "I AM TRYING TO USE WILLPOWER." I get angry and then embarrassed that people can see my problem.

11. Despite evidence to the contrary, have you continued to assert that you can diet "on your own" whenever you wish?

I keep trying, but I haven't been able to diet, with or without the help of diet programs, in a very long time. Something is wrong with me—in no time, my mind strays off the goal, I lose sight of my vision and I overeat.

12. Do you crave to eat at a definite time, day or night, other than mealtime?

I think of eating all the time, but the desire is more intense mid-afternoons, when the children are napping, and late evenings, after my boys are settled in bed. I like to eat when I finally sit down and relax.

13. Do you eat to escape from worries or trouble?

I do not intentionally eat to escape from my troubles, but I do find myself overeating when I am worried. It seems to be a natural reaction for me.

14. Have you ever been treated for obesity or a food-related condition?

I have gone to doctors and nutritionists for help. Each time I was given a new and improved diet, and I was instructed to practice self-control. Maybe I need a psychologist—a doctor to help me handle my emotions. Maybe then I could control my overeating.

15. Does your eating behavior make you or others unhappy?

My eating behavior makes me very unhappy, and my family is affected by my low self-esteem. I am hurting myself, but I cannot stop. I don't know how to stop. I know God loves me and wants me to be happy. Why do I keep overeating when it makes me so unhappy? What is wrong with me? Something is definitely wrong with me.

Shine Little Glow Worm

Passing the test with flying colors, I qualified for the title, "Compulsive Overeater." It was an easy mark, A+, no doubt in my mind. I could have asked more questions or attended a meeting listed in the packet of information, but instead I harbored resentment and anger. For months, I blamed my upbringing, my husband and my circumstances for my sorry state of affairs. Mixed-up and confused, I continued my efforts to control my diet. I continued to fail. In time, I gave up.

Sobbing into my pillow after another awful day of overeating, I made the decision to attend a meeting "for curiosity's sake." Being an instigator and a saleswoman by nature, I dragged my cousin and my best friend along for the ride. They were eating buddies and diet-minded like me. It was an easy sale, a miracle cure. We all wanted to be thin, but had no idea how to stop overeating. Anxious for help, we found a meeting the next day. It was conveniently located at a local church hall.

I welcomed Saturday. The sun shone brightly through the beautiful blue sky. I gathered the troops and drove to the meeting. We walked into the building and followed the signs for the meeting location. As always, I led the way. At the far corner of a huge hall, people were arranging metal folding chairs in a circle. One of the stout women sauntered across the room to greet us. I assumed she could tell by our sizes that we were looking for a diet group. We introduced ourselves and settled into some seats close to the door. She smiled politely and whispered, "You have come to the right place."

Taking an unofficial head count, there were maybe twelve to fifteen men and women in the group, mostly young and middle-aged adults representing a wide scope of shapes and sizes. Some were bone thin, some were grossly obese and some were normal sized, appearing pretty healthy. *That's what I want. I wish that I could be normal sized and healthy.*

The meeting opened with the Serenity Prayer. My mother loved that prayer. She would mumble it whenever she needed help. It was like a quick release switch to soften life's dilemmas.

> God grant me the serenity to accept the things I cannot change, the courage to change the things I can, and the wisdom to know the difference. (Reinhold Niebuhr)

Peace, acceptance, courage and wisdom, how do I apply that to my overeating? I listened intently as the men and women talked about the changes that had occurred since joining the program. The most prevalent message was "I stopped compulsively overeating by practicing the program. Just like the recovering alcoholic stops drinking, I do it one day at a time." I was intrigued. My friends, on the other hand, were not pleased. I could tell they were disenchanted the moment we walked into that musty church basement. They wiggled in their seats, looked at me, looked at their watches every few minutes and looked at me again. Their unspoken words were written across their scowling faces, "Why did you bring us here?"

The meeting closed with the Lord's Prayer. I gathered some pamphlets from the literature table, and we left without saying a word to anyone. On the way out the door, my companions laughed at the "sick people" and vowed never to return. Feeling embarrassed by my own sickness, I remained silent. I needed to return. My life was at stake.

Glimmer, Glimmer

At home, I read and reread my pamphlets. In my dreams, I was one of those thin, healthy-looking women. Although I could not imagine life without occasionally overeating, I was ready to attend my second meeting. This time I traveled alone. As I entered the church hall, a kind-looking rather plump woman recognized me from the week before. She smiled meekly and said, "Welcome back." I felt an immediate bond as her sad eyes met mine. She told me about her week. I told her about mine. We were both out-of-control eaters. I did not intend to tell her what I did with food, but as she told me her tragic tale, it was easy to tell her my equally disheartening turn of events. We were like sisters, two peas in a pod. We smiled in hopeful anticipation as the beautiful speaker-of-the-day began her talk.

She was not an eloquent speaker by any means, nor was she particularly happy. As I saw it, she was just like me, crazy, always thinking about food and her weight, but there was a difference, a big difference, she was thin and was no longer overeating. The woman said, "Get a sponsor who has what you want and ask how she is achieving it." She looked good to me. I wanted to get thin. After the meeting, I bravely approached her. "Please, can you help me?"

She peered at me, acted rather perturbed and said, "Are you sure you are ready to give up sugar?" Evading the question, I explained that I was a newcomer to the program, but I was an informed dieter. I asked, "Could I follow a diet from Weight Watchers or Diet Workshop?" Disgruntled, she said either diet could work *if* I carefully refrained from sugar. I overlooked her unpleasant attitude and agreed sugar was certainly a problem for me.

After an anxious moment and a sigh, she apologized for her inconsiderate behavior and explained that she had a full plate. Many people called her during the day at prearranged times to commit their food. She seemed to force a smile and said, "Okay, we'll try it. Call me at 8 A.M. tomorrow, and tell me what you are going to eat for the day.

Driving home, I felt as if a giant boulder had been lifted off my shoulders. I had someone who was helping me. I had a group of people helping me. I was not alone anymore. The sun felt warmer, the sky seemed bluer, and life seemed better. A revelation hit me. It was a spiritual awakening of sorts. Twelve-step programs work because people share from the heart of experience. What a simple concept. *Thank you, God. My sponsor person might not be the most pleasant woman in the world, but whatever she is doing works for her. That's good enough for me.*

As I was nearing home, I wondered what to tell Carl. I was afraid of his reaction to yet another dieting scheme. He had already witnessed so many new diets, so many hopes, dreams and so many failures. My fear kept me silent. He didn't need to know the details. The proof would speak for itself. I quietly rummaged through my books and decided on a diet. I jotted down my intended plan for the next day. It was a funny state of mind; I was happy to have found my answer, but I was afraid. *No more cookies, no more cakes, no more cookie dough or frosting?* It only made sense to eat all the things I would never be able to eat again. I was kissing my goodies good-bye, so to speak. Although I knew I would feel physically full, it seemed okay this time. My life was going to change.

Starlight, Starbright

The next day I awoke eager to begin. I called my sponsor and told her what I was planning to eat for the day. Program jargon confused me. The word "abstinent" was in every sentence. I asked, "What does it mean to be abstinent?" "It is simple," she said, "Abstinence is refraining from compulsive overeating. When people say they have been abstinent for a year, it means they have followed their diet every single day for a whole year." That amazed me. How could anyone go a whole year without sugar? *That would be a miracle for me.* She went on to say that a sponsor is the person who helps you get started. She tells you what to do to achieve abstinence.

I was ready to receive my instructions: "Read a daily meditation book for addicts," and call other people who are in program. Ask them how they stay "out of the food." It was all new terminology. "We don't eat one day at a time." I asked, "What do you mean you don't eat?" She said, "We eat what we plan and nothing else. Some people do a 301 meal plan, three meals a day with nothing in between, except water or black coffee, one day at a time." My sponsor believed in a less restrictive approach. Any diet without sugar was fine. Nutritionally it made sense to me. We were off to a good start.

"Get a pencil and paper," she commanded. "I want you to jot down some telephone numbers. Keep them on the side of the refrigerator for easy reference." This woman knew lots of people and all their telephone numbers by heart. "You need to hear about compulsive overeating and how to stop when you get too hungry, angry, lonely or tired." She said, "We need to halt. Remember that word." The phone call concluded with one more question. "Can you make a commitment to attend a meeting every Saturday morning?" I told her I would try. "It might be difficult because my husband works a lot, and I have two small children." She understood and told me to go if I could.

It was Sunday morning, around 9 A.M., when I hung up the phone. Amazingly enough everyone in the house was still sleeping. Although I felt leery calling strangers, I had agreed to call one person sometime during the day. I took advantage of the free time and called the first person on my list. The first call went well. I felt compelled to call the next person and continued until I had called every person on my list. It was a new fun experience. People wanted to talk. They seemed happy to have gotten my call. Strangers wanted to help me. I sat in awe. All this advice was free. People helped people, just because people had helped them.

Somehow, I stayed on my diet for days, weeks and months. My weight dropped steadily, and I gathered strength, wisdom and understanding as I avoided sugar one day at a time. I learned to redirect my compulsive nature to helping other sick and suffering overeaters. I made phone calls, encouraged people and never said, "I can't help you." I had the answer, people helping people. Without sugar, it was easy to diet.

All That Glitters is Not Gold

Many people walked into our meeting never to return. It broke my heart. I had been given an extra measure of compassion for the discouraged overeater. My family and job sat on the back burner at this stage of my life. When the phone rang, I talked. I had a mission, save *all* the compulsive overeaters who needed help. Faithfully I attended the Saturday meeting. I shared my success story each week.

Being bold and outspoken, my reputation went before me: "She's a know-it-all." It fit me. My big-shot attitude kept me hopping from sponsor to sponsor. I did not listen well. I already had the answers. I felt that I had done my homework. My personal dieting experience, plus the oodles of books about nutrition that I had read, made me an expert or so I thought. I was certainly a whiz at food exchanges and calories.

As I continued in the program, my harshness softened, and I became a desirable sponsor. Knowing about nutrition was helpful in leading people to a healthy food plan. The list of people that I sponsored was long, too long. Coming from extremely low self-esteem, I reveled in being good at something.

Gradually I forgot about taking care of myself. I didn't have time to talk about me. I was busy helping everyone else. At one point, I was relieved when my "sponsor of the week" ate and decided to leave the program. I made the decision to sponsor myself. Why not? I was successful and I was thin. My sick thinking told me that my time would be better spent sponsoring other people. I was fine.

Without a sponsor, it was easy to make exceptions to the rules. I ate more than my plan allowed, usually additional protein, potato or rice. I forgave myself each time and decided I could not be perfect. I did not want to be perfect.

People talked about different food plans. Some people were successfully doing a food plan that sounded dreadful to me. It was called the "The Gray Sheet." I supposed that the original plan of eating must have been printed on a gray sheet of paper. It was a food plan that eliminated all grains. It certainly didn't appeal to me. I liked my grains. I couldn't imagine life without them. I ate oatmeal for breakfast; at lunch and dinner, I ate rice cakes, baked potato or some rice. I avoided bread because it was too fluffy. Although somewhere along the line, I made the decision that diet bread would be okay. It was an easy option. In time, I went to a nutritionist for more ideas. She suggested that a bagel or a muffin might add some variety. We discussed my goal to avoid sugar. She understood how junk food could be detrimental to my health, but convinced me that bagels and muffins were healthy exchanges.

One day I said, "Okay, I will buy some corn muffins." I had avoided sugar for nine months, but how much sugar could there be in one corn muffin? Empowered and confident, I felt the health factor would benefit me. It would be fine. I knew how to stay on my diet. I was abstinent from sugar, I was thin and I looked good. *I can do this. A corn muffin is a healthy food. I'll be fine.*

The big day came. I ate my corn muffin and I felt like a hero. Three days later, I bought six corn muffins and ate them in the car on the way home from the store. I was shocked at how fast the familiar pattern of compulsive overeating, followed by stringent dieting, returned. Embarrassed, I attended fewer meetings. Quietly sitting in my chair, my face revealed my pain. I lost my status and became a seeker once more.

I tried and tried to follow the same diet. I could do it for a few days, sometimes a week or a month, but then I would binge once more. Two years passed. I searched for the answer. People at the meetings told me that I had fallen off my pink cloud. Others told me I was doing more research. I was doing more pain, more compulsive overeating. People often say, "There is nothing worse than a belly full of food and a head full of program."

Follow the Yellow Brick Road

Somberly I waited for the meeting to begin. Empty and alone, I hung my head in shame. *What is wrong with me? I cannot make it through one day on my diet.* A tear trickled down my cheek. *Lord, please show me the way. I am so tired.* The day before my mother died, she was heavy-hearted and discouraged. She looked to the sky and reminisced. A comforting verse came to mind.

Jesus said, "Come to me, all you who are weary and burdened, and I will give you rest." (Matthew 11:28, *New International Version*)

Please, Lord, help me. What do You want me to do?

A radiant young woman volunteered to lead the meeting. Hope glistened in my heart when she described her transformed life. My heart skipped a beat when she explained her food plan, absolutely no sugar *or* flour. She boldly proclaimed, "My food plan is weighed and measured. Sugar *and flour* are no longer options for me."* *[The refinement process of whole grains into flour increases the absorption rate of these foods into the bloodstream. Only a tad slower than sugar, flour affects the serotonin levels in the brain. That's why we feel like sleeping after a binge of highly refined carbohydrates. Serotonin acts like a tranquilizer, a painkiller and an escape from life.]

I froze for a moment, does not compute, I could not comprehend that ghastly thought. *No flour?* I cringed. My heart ached. My mind spun in search of logic. I wanted to deny the validity of such drastic measures. *Come on, Lord, flour, too? Flour is healthy. My nutritionist told me breads and pastas are good foods.* My future was grim. I could not imagine life without flour, my muffins, my bagels, my "healthy" foods. I asked for an answer, some other answer, any other answer.

God whispered in my ear, "Can you do it for one day?" I stopped grumbling. *Maybe, just maybe, recovery is more complicated than I thought. Flour could be addictive. Sugar is certainly a problem for me.* It was a gruesome thought, but I was tired of living a miserable life. Gloom and doom had followed me for a very long time. This woman had celebrated five years of abstinence. She was thin *and* she was happy. She had a calm delight, an aura of godliness. I wanted that peace.

She volunteered to sponsor one new person, one *serious* person. She only helped people looking for *serious* recovery. I was desperate and I was tired of doing things my way. It didn't work. I remembered my first spiritual awakening months before. 12-steppers share from the heart of experience. This profound experience birthed my second spiritual awakening; *recovering* food addicts not only weigh and measure their food, but they avoid sugar *and* flour. My first phase in program was a diet. I had listened to Weight Watchers logic. I had gotten thin, looked successful and I felt good for a while. A diet is only a diet. Food addiction relates to specific foods known to set up cravings in the body of an

_____. God wanted me to understand the severity of the disease and the power of His help.

Jesus Gave Me a Sunbeam

"Please, let me be the one." Her twinkling eyes met my pleading spirit. She said, "That would be wonderful." My heart rejoiced. *Thank you, God.* It was as if a beam of sunshine landed on my shoulders and radiated its warmth all the way to my soul. My life changed as my wellspring of knowledge disappeared.

I surrendered my will, my wants, my intellect and my perceived know-how to her. She understood the intricacies of food addiction. She set the guidelines beginning with my diet. She gave me the basic plan that had been passed down the line of sponsors. The bottom line was absolutely no sugar and flour. She emphasized dependence on God.

"A successful life-changing program is more than following a food plan, so much more. It is a relationship with God." She said that my new life would start with self-control around my food, then God would use that experience to give me courage, strength and confidence to apply the 12-step principles in *all* my affairs. It was yet another awakening;

addiction recovery is a lifestyle change beyond getting thin. The 12-Step program is the map to lasting recovery.

"If you want what I have, do what I do." The rule still applied. "Quiet time is the most important time of the day." She told me to pray and meditate for thirty minutes in the morning. "It is the most important thing." She continued to explain that her program was modeled from Alcoholics Anonymous. "They work a life or death program. Alcohol is not an option for a recovering alcoholic, just like eating sugar and flour is not an option for a recovering food addict."

She told me that the Big Book is the resource for addiction recovery. It is tried and true. "Read it each day, one page at a time, starting with The Doctor's Opinion. Then I want you to read page 449, the page on acceptance and page 83, the promises of the program."

> We are going to know a new freedom and a new happiness. We will not regret the past nor wish to shut the door on it. (*Alcoholics Anonymous*, Third Edition, page 83)

She mentioned matter-of-factly that it might seem like a lot of work, but we need to put as much into our recovery as we put into our overeating. I must have looked dumbfounded, wide-eyed and opened-mouthed. It was fear,

fear of failure or was it fear of success? I had a Big Book, but had never read it from cover to cover, only bits and pieces now and then, usually to help me to understand Carl's problem.

She asked if I was still willing. "Do you want to rise above your addiction once and for all?" I nodded sheepishly making every attempt to hold back my tears and whimpered, "For one day at a time, right?" Her whole face smiled. She sweetly touched my hand. "Yes, dear, it is just one day at a time. Sometimes it's one hour, one minute, one second at a time." My oppression lifted. Hope flowed into my veins.

She continued to give me my instructions. "I want you to read the daily meditation from the *Twenty-Four Hours a Day* Book published by Hazelden. People call it 'the little black book.'" She told me to thank God for yesterday, ask Him for help today and paraphrase the first three steps in simple terms, "I am powerless over food, people, places and things. God can help me. I will let Him by turning my will and my life over to His care today." Then I was told to memorize the third-step prayer. "Say it whenever you feel like overeating. Learn one line at a time until it is an automatic response to a food thought."

God I offer myself to Thee—to build with me and do with me as Thou wilt. Relieve me of the bondage of self, that I may better do Thy will. Take away my difficulties, that victory over them may bear witness to those I would help of Thy power, Thy love, and Thy Way of Life. May I do Thy will always! (*Alcoholics Anonymous*, Third Edition, page 63)

Her final words encouraged me the most, "I'll pray for you, and you pray for me." This was a new ball game, so to speak. I was ready to hit a home run. On July 23, 1988, new life started to emerge. I had more than hope. I had skills to succeed one day at a time. I envisioned a caterpillar growing inside his cocoon. One day it would fly away as a beautiful butterfly, free at last.

Dawn's Early Light

The alarm rang. It was 6 A.M., my first day of abstinence. I fell to my knees and prayed for the willingness to see and do God's will. I gathered my books and read my page of the Big Book, The Doctor's Opinion. I was awestruck. My mind and heart saw the doctor's words cleverly confirming my personal revelations. For me as a food addict, excess food, sugar and flour are just as alcohol is to the alcoholic.

The only relief we have to suggest is entire abstinence. (*Alcoholics Anonymous*, Third Edition, page xxviii)

Okay, Lord, I get it. I am not weird or crazy. I have a disease. I have a sickness. I need my medicine. I need to abstain from sugar, flour and excessive quantities, and I need to depend on You, Lord, for help. I know this is the truth. There is no other way for me. I tried it all. This is the end of the line. The choice is life or death. I choose life.

My friends and family members continued to coerce me into believing a little self-control was my cure. Acceptance of myself as a food addict with all its peculiarities, was necessary. People do not need to understand the intricacies of the addicted body and mind, but the addict needs a sure foundation of the truth. Namely, we are different from the normal eater. It is okay. We have a disease.

The delusion that we are like other people, or presently may be, has to be smashed... (*Alcoholics Anonymous*, Third Edition, page 30.)

I made a commitment to do an in-depth study of the Twelve Steps with a group of serious, abstinent people, and I continued to read the Big Book to gain more understanding about the cunning and baffling aspects of addiction. I directed my attention to *my* attitudes, *my* responses and *my* responsibilities. I stopped blaming people, places and things for my trials and tribulations. I found strength and wisdom in understanding God's will for my life.

> Rarely have we seen a person fail who has thoroughly followed our path. Those who do not recover are people who cannot or will not completely give themselves to this simple program... (*Alcoholics Anonymous*, Third Edition, page 58)

Progress, Not Perfection

I stood at the threshold of my new life. My impression of the steps was basic, but powerful. God opened my eyes to dig deeper as I got stronger.

Step one: We admitted we were powerless over our food addiction—that our lives had become unmanageable.

I admitted that I was out of control. No matter how hard I tried, I could not stop overeating. In 12-step halls, I heard, "self-will run riot." My overeating was destroying my health and my relationships with family, friends and even God. I was spiraling downhill fast. My life was falling apart.

Step two: Came to believe that a power greater than ourselves could restore us to sanity.

I believed in God's love and His ability to restore me, but I needed to learn new coping skills. Therefore, the "power greater than myself" was the group of people who were living free from food obsession and overeating one day a time. I was hopeful. What God did for them, He could do for me.

Step three: Made a decision to turn our will and our lives over to the care of God as we understood Him.

I gave up. "Let go and let God" is the slogan that goes hand-in-hand with this step. I let go of my old way of doing things, and I started listening, learning and living in the solution. IE: I became a dedicated and committed 12-stepper. Practicing the tools became an integral part of my life. Meetings, phone calls, literature—especially reading the Big Book—committing my food plan to a sponsor, love and service, anonymity, writing were all instrumental in my forward surge. When I turned my will and my life over to God, my whole world changed—physically, emotionally and spiritually.

Step four: Made a searching and fearless moral inventory of ourselves.

Initially, the fifteen questions from the newcomer's kit revealed my sorry state of affairs. When I committed to 12-

step work, I kept my secrets, thoughts and feelings in a daily journal.

Step five: Admitted to God, to ourselves, and to another human being the exact nature of our wrongs.

God and I knew that I had problems. That was easy. The hard part was admitting to another person that I had a warped relationship with food. I talked to my cousin and my friend, which was a beginning. In program, I talked to friends at meetings and on the telephone, and I talked to my new sponsor. I soon learned that I was not alone.

Step six: Were entirely ready to have God remove all these defects of character.

In Step Six, the head connects to the heart. My head had to be convinced that my heart knew best. I wanted to follow God (my heart), but my self-control and defiant nature were deeply rooted in my dysfunctional lifestyle (my head).

Step seven: Humbly asked Him to remove our shortcomings.

I became willing to say, "I can't, You can, Please help me, God."

Step eight: Make a list of all persons we had harmed and became willing to make amends to them all.

My husband and my boys were first on my list, plus myself. Yes, there were others, but I couldn't see beyond my immediate family until I cleaned up my side of the street at home.

Step nine: Made direct amends to such people wherever possible, except when to do so would injure them or others.

I faced my fears and apologized to Carl for all the selfish, self-centered ways that I put food before his needs. Dan and Joe were young children, but I sat them down and asked their forgiveness. It was simple-stated truth at a level that they understood. The hardest person to face was myself. Acceptance that I was not perfect, and I would never be perfect this side of heaven, was an incredible revelation for me. The act of seeking forgiveness and being forgiven lightened my heart and brought me an element of peace that I had never known before.

Step ten: Continued to take personal inventory, and when we were wrong promptly admitted it.

I worked the program one day at a time. Praying for God's will, I practiced the tools to the best of my ability. At the end of each day, I got on my knees again and reviewed my day. I asked God what I needed to do in order to stay free (physically, emotionally and spiritually). If I lost my temper, made a snide remark or acted inappropriate in some way during the day, I'd apologize. Verbal utterance was good, but amending the behavior for the future was better. My relationship with God improved each time I called on His ever-available help.

Step eleven: Sought through prayer and meditation to improve our conscious contact with God *as we understood Him*, praying only for knowledge of His will for us and the power to carry that out.

Prayer is asking. Meditating is listening. My conversations with God increased when I surrendered to the disease. What choice did I have? Alone I could do nothing. It didn't take long for me to realize that with God I could do what seemed impossible. My humble prayers worked.

Step twelve: Having had a spiritual awakening as the result of these steps, we tried to carry this message to food addicts, and to practice these principles in all our affairs.

I carried the torch. God blessed me with an amazing gift—freedom from compulsive overeating and food obsession. It was a miracle of sorts. Sharing my experience, strength and hope was a privilege and a joy.

Chapter Four

Action—A Work in Progress

"Trust in the Lord with all your heart and lean not
on your own understanding; in all your ways
acknowledge him, and he will make your paths
straight."

(Proverbs 3:5-6, New International Version)

Baby Steps

The 12-step program is not "religious," but it *is* a
spiritual journey. The recovering addict is restored,
rejuvenated and revived to physical and emotional health
through trust and confidence in a spiritual connection with
"a higher power." When we surrender, we begin the process
of letting go of our attempts to control our environment.
Accepting that there is "a higher power" is a baby step
toward finding and knowing God.

Food addicts surrender to a food plan through the help of recovering food addicts. We humbly admit that we tried to stop overeating by stringent resolves to diet repeatedly, but we failed. Each time we fell on our faces, we were more frustrated and more desperate. When we gave up, recovering food addicts helped us to see that we have a physical, emotional and spiritual malady. In time, we see God, *as we understand Him*, working in our lives.

I have witnessed awesome transformations where the light of God's glory opened the eyes of people who were blinded by hurt, anger and resentment. Slowly, little awakenings, casual thoughts and realizations, touch the hearts of the skeptics. As they remain abstinent day after day, negative thinking dissipates as positive, life-giving strength flows in. They learn to "let go and let God" in everything.

> This is the how and why of it. First of all, we had to quit playing God. It didn't work. Next, we decided that hereafter in this drama of life, God was going to be our Director. He is the Principal; we are His agents. He is the Father, and we are His children. Most good ideas are simple, and this concept was the keystone of the new and triumphant arch through which we pass to freedom. (*Alcoholics Anonymous*, Third Edition, page 62)

First Things First

Grocery list in hand, I gathered my gumption and walked into the grocery store quivering in fear. History is history. How many times had I walked into a marketplace fully intending to buy the right foods for my diet of the day? How many times did the sight of some scrumptious temptation tantalize my taste buds? In the blink of an eye, I would choose to wait one more day and splurge one more time.

Today is different. I have a choice. Life or death and I choose life. Please, God, help me buy only the foods I need today. I can't do this alone. Give me the strength and willingness to ignore the aisles of junk foods. I need to focus my attention on this new diet, oh, I mean "food plan." I am not on a diet anymore. This is a way of life, a lifestyle change.

Oat bran, oatmeal and rice... my grocery list began. Easy enough, I found the boxes and bags without a hitch. Lots of vegetables and some fruits... I marched to the fresh produce department. My mouth began salivating when I spied the delectable rosy red apples. Carefully inspecting the biggest, most beautiful ones, I placed my exquisite find in a plastic bag and cradled it in the palm of my hand. *If I only get one apple, it's going to be luscious.*

Potatoes were next on my list. I loved the robust flavor of russet potatoes. The hearty skins were chewy, and the inners were firm and solid, more money for your buck, so to speak. I rummaged through the raunchy selection. Asking the store clerk for help, he went to the storeroom and brought out another pile to add to the slim pickings. I found my prize in a gorgeous, brunette beauty, probably ten or twelve ounces, no word of a lie. I tossed some salad fixings into my carriage, grabbed some carrots and proceeded to the condiments.

Not expecting much of a response, I approached the little girl stocking the shelves. "Do you know where I could find a low-calorie salad dressing without sugar or artificial sweetener? She shrugged her shoulders as if to say, "I don't know and I don't care." My diet mentality wanted it all, no calories, no sugar, no artificial sweetener.

I began my hunt for the perfect salad dressing. It was mission impossible. After examining label after label, I reluctantly succumbed to the truth that every low-calorie, low-fat salad dressing had one "no-no" or another. I settled for Paul Newman's Original. It was not low in calories, but it was free from sugar and artificial sweetener, and the proceeds were contributed to a good cause. I closed the door on that subject and moved to the next item on my list.

Plain yogurt... *sounds like swamp food to me. If I can find one with fruit and no sugar or artificial sweetener, that will be good enough.* Scouring the labels on each container, I was determined to find one that would fit the bill. No luck. Another surrender. *Plain yogurt will be fine. My sponsor said that it is only food, like gas for the tank of my car. I wonder if I'll ever feel that way.*

Only a few more things left to buy... chicken, eggs, ground beef, and tuna. It was a simple stroll down the refrigerator aisle with a slight detour to grab the tuna. I was ready to check out. As I worked my way to the front of the store, I picked up a few groceries for the family.

My sponsor's words warbled in my head. ***My food is my food and everything else is not my food. It is not an option to overeat, no matter what is happening in my circumstances or how I feel.*** On purpose, I chose a check out line free from temptations. With a bold sense of accomplishment, I paid for my food and sauntered out the door elated. *I did it...we did it. Thank you, God.* Willingness replaced my defiance. Faith replaced my fear.

Easy Does It

"Sunshine on my shoulders makes me happy." *Yes, John Denver, I concur.* With a leap in my step and joy in my heart, I jumped out of bed raring to go. I put the coffee on and fell to my knees in humble adoration and gratitude. "Lord, thank you, thank you, thank you. I will be forever grateful. You have answered my prayer." With a sly smile and a chuckle, I tacked on, "Why did You wait so long?" Then I continued, "I know...You know what You're doing. I am stubborn, but I am listening today."

The sun was shining, for me anyway. The toasty warm brilliance felt as if God had wrapped His loving arms around my entire being. Joy filled me to the brim.

It was 8 A.M., time to call my sponsor. My food plan was simple, The 301 Plan, three meals a day with nothing in between, except black coffee, tea or water, one day at a time.

Breakfast:	One serving of oatmeal or oat bran, 1 cup of plain yogurt and a fruit
Lunch:	½ cup protein, 1 cup cooked vegetables, 2 cups salad with 1 T. salad dressing
Dinner:	Same as lunch with one addition—a potato or 1/2 cup of rice

I poured my coffee, splashed a little milk in it and dialed the number. *I don't think a little milk could hurt. It's not sugar or flour. Milk is okay.* It took two seconds to report my food. My heart started palpating. Swallowing my self-sufficiency, I peeped, "Is it okay if I dribble a tad of skim milk in my coffee?" She retorted most emphatically, "The plan is three meals a day with *nothing* in between. Milk is food." The words were like daggers piercing my heart. My spine arched; my intentions hung in the air. Somberly I bid her farewell and hung up the phone.

I stared at my half-finished cup of coffee. *She is over the edge, maybe even crazy. Skim milk only has 80 calories in a whole cup.* God entered the scene with His sympathetic spirit and nudged me ever so gently, "Can you do it for one day?" Still negotiating, I muttered, "Maybe."

Angrily I opened my Big Book to Chapter Five, How It Works. I read about surrender, needing help, needing God. Then it came to me:

> Half measures availed us nothing. We stood at the turning point. We asked His protection and care with *complete* abandon." (*Alcoholics Anonymous*, Third Edition, page 59)

"Okay, Lord, I will give you my milk, too, but I'm not happy about it."

Amusingly enough, my coffee tasted more enticing and better than ever. It took three gulps before I professed, "This will be okay. I like it. I can do this." I had hurdled my first obstacle, and I didn't die. I fell to my knees and said, "Thank you, God."

Bump in the Road

Our mini-van was strategically packed with cooler, grill, special cooking supplies and the usual bags and baggage. We were ready to roll. One amazing week of abstinence under my not-so-tight belt, I faced my first vacation without food. As I adjusted my seat belt, I drifted into a trance, totally engrossed in self-pity. *What am I going to do for a whole week at the beach?* Vacations were supposed to be fun. *How in the world do you have fun without food?* It was a mystery to me.

Carl and the boys loved the beach. Dan was eight and Joe was six at the time. We had vacationed near the ocean every year since before the children were born. It was tradition. With joyful anticipation, Carl engaged the boys in conversation. I faked a smile. They reminisced about their walks on the beach, the sand castles, the fishing and the food. I contributed nothing. Vacations were all about eating in my book.

As we traveled from one town to the next, Dan and Joe munched on their packets of travel supplies. Little bags of penny candy kept them occupied and content until we reached our first milestone. "Are we at McDonald's yet, Mommy? I'm hungry." Daniel began. Carl grumbled disgustedly, "You are just like your mother, eating in wait for your next meal." My eyes rolled towards the sky and I mumbled, "Lord, help me." They had learned from the master. I wished things were different. *Carl is right. The boys are just like me. God bless them.*

After a moment of pity and sadness for the boys and myself, I announced, "I can't change yesterday, but I can change today." Carl's disbelieving eyes darted in my direction as if to say, "I've heard that before." I was not credible. My words held empty promises for too many years. It didn't matter. At that moment, his nonverbal conviction hurt. Feeling perturbed, I proclaimed, "This time is different."

Poor Carl. I was a tough cookie to deal with, a pandemonium of fear and insecurity. I was up one minute and down the next. Just a simple misunderstood look would force him to run for cover. I never physically threw things or hurt anyone, but my eyes shot daggers, and my words and body language could be dismal. To say I was "temperamental" would be polite.

After Carl's hurtful glance, we sat in silence while I tried to gather my composure. *Lord, help me. I want to have a fun vacation with the family.* We pulled into the parking lot of McDonald's. My dinner was ready and waiting in my new, carefully chosen compact cooler with my hand-picked, color-coordinated plastic containers. Carl laughed when he eyed my precision custom packing job. I laughed with him. I was not insulted this time. It was comical and a tad over the edge. I had spent a good amount of time obsessing over the perfect travel gear for my new way of life. It appeased me somehow to have special equipment. My sponsor said that I needed to spend as much time in recovery as I had in the disease. This year I bought supplies instead of food. It was a big step for me to pack my meal and then actually eat it. The Big Mac's looked mighty appealing.

The vacation was not fun. I walked and talked, but wanted to crawl out of my skin. On every corner and every side street, I saw someone eating something. All my favorite vacation foods were dancing in the air, singing an inviting chant, "Just have one. You're on vacation. You deserve to have fun."

One minute at a time, I resisted the temptation. In moments of surrender, I stopped to feel the sunshine on my shoulders, and I thanked God. More often, I was agitated and downright angry. *Why do I have this disease*? I hoped for relief. People told me it would come in God's time. Trying to look on the bright side, I decided to approach the vacation as a challenge, an opportunity to practice my program.

The Jury is Out

"Baby, you're no fun anymore," Carl complained. Fun to us meant eating, sometimes at nice restaurants, sometimes here, there and everywhere, strolling along the beach, camping in front of the fire, a drive to get ice cream, take-out with a movie at home. Even though my husband was not a compulsive overeater like me, he *was* most assuredly an eating buddy of mine.

The day arrived when he lovingly suggested that we go out to dinner. I cringed and suggested that he order take-out, pizza or Chinese food. "I'll be happy to pick it up and bring it home." Trying to encourage him to consider the advantages,

I added, "You can unwind, kick off your shoes and get comfortable." My ulterior motive—I could then have my planned food. He rolled his eyes in dismay. It was as if he needed his dance partner. We all know you can't dance alone, slow dancing anyway. He wanted his bosom buddy to come home.

In those first few months of abstinence, my poor husband was kicked aside like a worn-out shoe. My experienced counterpart was no longer needed. It took every ounce of effort for me to survive without overeating. My sponsor told me to stick to my guns, "Do not go out to dinner until you have at least three months of abstinence." I conveyed her words to Carl. He was angry. "What makes her your boss?" I was a basket case full of confusion, wanting recovery, but wondering about the cost. I prayed for my answer.

Carl tried to listen to my explanation. I was afraid that I might overeat. It was as if I were talking to a wall. Carl was not like me. Only another food addict knows the devastation and pain I feel when my disease rears its ugly head, and you never know when it will appear. Time was like insurance or money in the bank. I was hoping for a stretch of confident abstinence before I was forced to step into the ring with my disease.

Tough as it was to defy my sponsor, I surrendered to my husband, and we set a date. The fight began, my desire for more food versus my desire for recovery, tough competitors. It was good versus evil, so to speak. My sponsor wasn't happy, but she told me what to do: "Cut the meat to the size of a deck of cards. Order a baked potato and two salads. Eat one salad as an appetizer and the other with the meal. Bring your salad dressing, or have two teaspoons oil and vinegar. Most meals come with a cooked vegetable. You can eat it *if* it was prepared without sugar or flour. Remember the bottom line is always no sugar or flour, no gravy, no sauces, no fancy vegetables, no fancy anything."

I said "okay" at the time, but when push came to shove, I changed my mind. *Lord, I'm not doing that. Abstinence is having a plan and doing the plan. I'll plan to order a meal free from sugar or flour, but I'll eat what I am served. I'll commit my plan to God. I'll be fine.* We put on our Sunday clothes, got a baby-sitter for the boys and slipped away. Our favorite restaurant had lots of variety. I ordered a prime rib, baked potato, the green beans, and two salads. I ate every bite. When the waitress asked if I was done, my husband said with a snicker, "She decided not to eat the plate." Sounds funny now, but at the time I was not amused.

I felt as if I had done well. I stopped when the meal was over. I refrained from sugar and flour, and I didn't eat any of the good stuff, no bread, pasta or desserts. It was healthy, abstinent food. *This is fun. It's like the date nights we had before we were married.* Minutes went by. My stomach started to hurt. *I ate too much. If I overeat every time I go out, I'll never get thin. My sponsor always says that abstinence is the most important thing without exception. I was abstinent. I did what I planned. I'll get thin in God's time.*

"Carl, when can we go out to dinner again?" I asked as we exited the parking lot of the restaurant. "That was fun." Carl was delighted that I had enjoyed our time together. He suggested that we go every Saturday night. This began my new preoccupation, my obsession of the week. I scoured every local newspaper, the telephone book and all the local flyers looking for the perfect place for our dinner date on Saturday night. I was being a good wife spending time with my husband and making him happy. Don't you agree?

Restaurant dining became an anticipated delight. Buffets were first-rate, top-notch, the cream of the crop, so to speak. My commitment sounded good on paper: one plate of food, two plates of salad and no good stuff, no sugar or flour, no coleslaw, no marinated vegetables, no sauces or gravies, no hard cheese. I brought my salad dressing.

Each time I went out to dinner, I wanted to be reasonable. I intended to be reasonable. More times than not, I would march to the food court, heap my one plate to embarrassing proportions with lots of meat, a mound of potatoes and a pile of vegetables. Then I would get my salads. I often complained about "the dinky salad plates." Pieces of my salads would topple off the overloaded heaps. My husband once commented, "You know, Baby, you can go to the buffet line as many times as you want. You don't have to stack all the food on one plate." My piercing eye shot him dead. I wanted to yell, "SHUT UP!" Guilt-ridden, I kept silent. I was feeding the disease by overeating and justifying it. *I deserved to have a good time with my husband. Abstinence is planning what you do and doing what you plan. I was abstinent. Right, Lord?*

Mama Mia

"Another meeting? This is ridiculous. Saturday, Tuesday and now Thursday! Don't those cronies know you have a life?" Carl's anger spouted forth in a wave of dismay.

It hit me. I cowered for a second, shrugged my shoulders, and I looked to the sky with a "please help me" plea. Sucking in my breath, I sighed one of those long, exasperating moans. I picked myself up and continued telling him what he could do for the boys, while I attended my meeting. "There is popcorn for the boys. Their pajamas are on the bench. If you want, I'll put them to bed when I get home."

"Mama, please don't go. *I need you* to help me with my homework," Dan begged as he dragged his book bag into the room, heavy from the amount of work he needed to accomplish.

"Mama, I don't feel good." My poor sad little one climbed on my lap and held me hostage for a minute.

Surprised and disappointed, the family heard, "I'm sorry guys, but I have to go. I love you." I walked out the door. As I looked back, Dan and Joe's faces were glued to the window. Somberly their dejected little expressions cried out, "How could you leave us?" I suspect they wondered what had happened to their mother. I blew them a kiss from the car and I started to cry. By the time I reached the end of our street, I was sobbing uncontrollably. I parked on the side of the road and let God calm me for a spell. I was still whimpering as I walked into my third meeting of the week.

First things had to come first, program, then family, then job. Abstinence is the most important thing without exception. Acceptance is the answer to all my problems today. Please, Lord, help me.

Life, as I had known it, was over. My lifelong ideas and concepts had been turned upside down. Placing myself and my needs before my family was beyond reason. *My children come first. They always have. They always will.* Learning that I was not neglecting them by taking care of myself, took time and lots of practice. It was not selfish and self-centered, as I had once thought.

Balancing Act

"Professional caretaker," that's me in a nutshell. Not only was taking care of people my paid job as a daycare provider for children, it was my passion and my heart's desire. I still love-to-love people, but now I do it in a balanced, constructive way with clear motives. Years ago, my goals were undefined beyond being the best wife, mother and daycare provider in the whole wide world, whatever it took.

Dan and Joe were the loves of my life. I spent hour after hour researching how to be the best parent possible. Determined to shower them with motherly affection, I coddled them beyond their needs. In retrospect, it was my attempt to protect them. I wished I could have placed them in a giant bubble where they could ride through life sheltered from the trials and tribulations of the world.

My job as wife held a close second in the line of priorities. Carl needed me. He was doing well in his new job. That was his identity. I felt that it was my responsibility to take care of the house and home, to clean, to cook and handle all the needs of the children. How could I go to a meeting and still do my job?

I tried. It was tough for me, but I was willing to practice. It was progress, not perfection. My sponsor implied I was soft. She said that I had a warped perception of family responsibilities and an overdeveloped sense of responsibility. She said I needed to let go and ask for help. "Carl is a big boy and the father of your children. He can handle a couple of hours at home alone with the boys. They are seven and nine, certainly not babies." She was right, but so was I. Sometimes my family needed me more than I needed a meeting. Other times I needed to go. When I felt like I was deserting the ship, I trusted God to protect, nurture and love my family.

Ruffled Feathers

It was 7:03 A.M. Tossing and turning in my rumpled bed, I could hear the clock ticking like a steady drip of water tapping on a tin roof, tick, tick, tick. *What am I going to say to my sponsor today? She will be miffed. I told her I was going to the meeting last night and then I didn't go. I'm in big trouble. I need to think of a good story, if I call* her at all. *The truth is the truth. I had every intention of going to the meeting, but Carl came home exhausted after working a tedious twelve-hour shift and poor Joe was sick again, wheezing up a storm. Asthma is scary. I stayed home to monitor his breathing.*

Thank God, we didn't end up at the hospital again. Lord, was I wrong? I didn't overeat, although a bagel or a doughnut would hit the spot right now. I know that that would be dumb. No way am I going back to that life. Please, Lord, what should I do? I rolled out of bed and dropped to my knees. Instinctively, I heard:

> Give all your worries and cares to God, for he cares about what happens to you. Be careful! Watch out for attacks from the Devil, your great enemy. He prowls around like a roaring lion, looking for some victim to devour. Take a firm stand against him, and be strong in your faith... (1 Peter 5:7-9, *New Living Translation*)

God, I know You were with me last night. I made the right decision to stay home. Whatever my sponsor thinks or feels about me is none of my business. God bless her. I picked up the phone and quickly dialed the number.

I was tempted to say, "I'm out of here, no woman is going to tell me that I should have gone to a meeting when my child is sick." Instead, I bit my tongue and tactfully explained my circumstances for another day. Yes, my sponsor felt I could have left Joe with Carl. It was okay. I had done the right thing. As she complained, I mumbled under my breath, "Oh well. God bless her." When she stopped talking, I told her what I was planning to eat for the day.

I learned that sponsors were perfectly imperfect people. Sponsors can only share up to the level of their experience. They are not professionals, simply volunteers *trying* to help another food addict get well. I have seen and tried to work with different types of sponsors in the program, everyone type from the rigid drill sergeants appearing insensitive, judgmental and controlling, to the laid-back insecure ones who are tossed and turned by the wind. They want to help, but don't have the skills or knowledge to succeed, no less teach it to someone else.

Sometimes it is a real blind leading the blind scenario. It is rare to find successful middle ground, but it is possible. Through trial, error and perseverance, we find the answers to our personal quest: What do I need to do to stop overeating one day at a time?

Queen of Hearts

My sponsor was an older woman with grown children. She could not relate to the demands and obligations of a young wife, mother and daycare provider. Her answer to any problem was "Go to more meetings." My life was full. For me, going to three meetings a week was nearly an impossible mission. When I skipped a meeting, regardless of the reason, I got the third degree. The gun barrel pointed to my head, she would say, "Why didn't you go?" If she disagreed with my decision, the lecture would follow; you know those talks where you hold the phone away from your ear, hand on your hip, waiting for the last line? I was her captive. When she released the prisoner, that's how I felt when she finally stopped talking, I would hang up the phone feeling spanked like a disobedient child.

I soon realized that my sponsor acted like me with my children. She was like an overprotective mother. She tried to control me just as I tried to control my children. I remember one day in particular. My Dan was only eight years old. It was one of those cold winter months in New England. Glistening snow gracefully danced in the air. The radio stationed announced, "Temperatures dropping to the teens today, snow on the way." Dan was getting ready for school. Our usual debate began. "Mom, I don't need my winter coat today." Calmly I began, "Please, Dan, it's going to be cold today." Back and forth we went, our voices escalating with each sentence. After a tad of bickering, I took his face in my hand, as I often did when I was frustrated and wanted his full attention. I squeezed his cheeks together, pointed his face in the direction of my words and I said without question, "You need your jacket today. Put it on."

When school was over, he hopped off the bus anxious to tell me about his day. Happily bounding into the house, he met my insensitive glare. Loudly I bellowed, "I told you to wear your coat! What is wrong with you?" He stopped in his tracks. His little puppy-dog eyes glazed over instantly. Jolted by rejection and disappointment, he gasped. Meekly, he uttered, "But, Mom, I wasn't cold." *What did that have to do with it?* Was I being unreasonable or do *good children obey their parents?*

If Dan were cold, he had a jacket to warm h[...] responsibility as his mother was to supply the coat, teach him to take care of himself and let God do the rest. My job as a person committed to recovery is to listen to program guidance, ask God for help and then make self-nurturing decisions according to the situations at hand. I wished my sponsor would make suggestions in kind, loving and respectful ways, but it was not her style.

Drawing the line between reasonable love and care for the family and my own needs of support and encouragement was difficult. It was trial and error. Some days I would stay home instead of going to a meeting. It was a wrong choice. I didn't slide into overeating, but the ground was slippery. It was only by the grace of God that I was able to sit on my hands or pull the sheets over my head some days to avoid incredible temptations. Through my own experiences, I became more aware of my emotional triggers and it was easier to accept my misconstrued motives. I didn't always agree with my sponsor's advice, but I listened and I grew stronger as each day passed.

Brokenhearted

"DANIEL, WHAT ARE YOU DOING?" I yelled at the top of my lungs. My poor Daniel looked petrified. It was the umpteenth time that I had raised my voice that day. *Why was I so angry?* Disappointed and confused, I collapsed on the couch sobbing. I wanted to crawl up into a ball and die. *What is wrong with me? Why am I so cruel?* True, he had made a mess in the kitchen. However, it was certainly not a punishable offense, nor were the other incidents cause for great alarm. Trying to practice my program, I apologized once again. It was embarrassing to say the same thing over and over again, but I did it anyway. "I'm sorry that I yelled at you. I will try to say what I mean, but not say it mean."

Dan wrapped his sweet little arms around my neck and tenderly replied, "It's okay, Mommy, I know you love me." My heart melted. I hugged him mercilessly, not wanting to let him go and thanked God for my precious children.

I called my sponsor and told her my problem, "Even though I keep trying, I cannot stop yelling!" She told me to go to more meetings. "Get out of the house" was her advice. Going to another meeting was not a viable option for me. I was already struggling with my commitment to attend three meetings a week. It was tough. Typically, I'd return to a madhouse. My husband had little patience with the boys. Almost instantaneously, as I walked through the door, I'd drink in the chaos and I'd think, "Give me something to eat."

Extra food was not a choice, so I got angry and resentful instead, which caused more yelling. Discouraged, I sank into a depression.

Lord, help me. I am so discouraged. I thought if I stopped overeating, I would be happy. I am not happy. What do You want me to do? I felt a quickening in my heart, "Don't give up before the miracle happens for you." A minute went by and the phone rang. One of my friends in program was gleaming. She had found a professional counselor who was helping her understand her unique challenges. "It's personal," she said, "We are not all the same. We have different backgrounds and individual struggles." I followed her lead, called the number, and set up my first appointment.

Help is on the Way

My calendar was marked in red, Thursday at 5:00 P.M. In preparation for our first session, the counselor suggested writing in a journal "to see if a pattern emerged." I bought a notebook and started scribbling some thoughts each day. Finally, it was time for my first appointment. Pacing in the waiting room, my anxiety rose. I stared at the hands on the clock above the door as the moments rolled slowly by.

When the receptionist finally called my name, I was "armed and dangerous." I barreled through the door firing my first question as we found our seats, "How many meetings should I attend?" It took a minute for him to speak. I think I knocked the wind out of him. Calmly and quietly, in his gentle and melodious voice, he began to teach me lifestyle remedies. "It is a personal decision. Many people do well with three meetings a week in the beginning. It depends on where you are with your food. If you feel as if you are going to eat, then you need to be at a meeting. Abstinence is the most important thing. When people say, "program, family, job," they mean abstinence first, that is freedom from obsession and the action that manifests from it." His voice calmed my raging spirit. I heard every word as it drifted into the room on a wave of serenity. I marveled at his peaceful state. I had come to the right place.

He went on to explain how some people replace life with meetings and it becomes the new obsession. However, he was very clear to point out that there is a transitional stage, where an addict learns how to live. "An addict needs to learn how to live without turning to his or her drug of choice." Going to meetings, working the steps, listening to other people who are like-minded are all tools to fix sick thinking. I remember his words even today, "Why don't you be an example of a food addict who learns how to live outside the meetings?" "Okay," I said with my determined spirit. "That will be my goal."

My psychologist understood addictions and encouraged me to continue my 12-step work. As I continued to attend my committed meetings each week, I could see God's hand in my life. The promises were more tangible, even for a low-bottom addict, like me.

> We will intuitively know how to handle situations which used to baffle us. We will suddenly realize that God is doing for us what we could not do for ourselves. (*Alcoholics Anonymous*, Third Edition, pages 84)

The Real Deal

"Look in the mirror and say what?" My counselor replied, "Look in the mirror and say, 'I am beautiful. I love you.'" Not for me. With much prodding, I stood in front of the mirror and painfully succumbed to the idea, "I'm okay. Jesus loves me." That was the best I could do. I tried to imagine liking myself more, even loving myself, but not for today. I had invested years in believing I was fat and unattractive. Therefore, I was unlovable. He gave me my instructions, "Whenever you hear yourself saying those negative words, replace them with the truth, 'I'm okay. Jesus loves me.' In time, with lots of practice, you will be saying, 'I am beautiful. I love you.' It is time to start replacing self-debasing lies with positive, life-giving truths."

"If you were to die today, what do you wish people would say about you?" Cunningly, I replied, "She was thin." Agitated, he repeated the question with emphasis. "What would you want people to say about you?" My smile left. I imagined my funeral with people milling around. After some uncomfortable silence and careful consideration, I concluded, "I would like to hear 'She was healthy and took care of herself. She was a kind and loving person. She was a wonderful wife, mother and daycare provider.'" His smile and approving nod indicated I understood the question.

He jotted my words on his pad. Searching for the truth, he said, "Do you believe you are a kind and loving person?" Embarrassed, I nodded my head. I hesitated for a second to contemplate the full picture. Then I admitted more adamantly, "Yes, my heart is kind and loving, *but* my mouth and attitude do not always reflect my compassionate spirit. I am angry and resentful, and I yell at my children much more than I'd like to admit. What is wrong with me, doctor?" He said, "Out of the heart the mind speaks. You will learn new skills. In time you will actually feel deserving of the title, *kind and loving.*" Wow, huh? My broken heart felt the healing touch of hope.

He gave me an assignment, to "Write it until you believe it." *I am a kind and loving person. I am a kind and loving person. I am a kind and loving person. I am okay; Jesus loves me. I am okay; Jesus loves me. I am okay; Jesus loves me.* It sounded strange and a waste of time, but I said, "Okay, I'll do it." Today, years later, I can honestly tell you, "I *am* a kind and loving person. I *am* beautiful in God's eyes and I *know* Jesus loves me."

Self-esteem rises as we acknowledge our feelings and our own dysfunctional thinking. *Feelings are not facts.* Self-confidence and God-reliance comes when self-centered lies dissolve. It was time to separate fact from fiction. My counselor asked, "Do you *react* to what you think, want or feel, or do you *respond* to the facts and what you know?" I didn't have a clue. He said, "With God's help, you will learn to respond to the truth." He gave me some examples. I have listed a few that are relevant in my life.

I think I am recovered from my eating disorder (lie); *I know* recovery is contingent on working the program one day at a time (truth).

I think I am alone. No one loves me. I am unlovable (lie); *I know* I am never alone. Jesus loves me, and He has made me in his image—lovable (truth).

I want to be normal. *I want* something to eat (unhealthy thinking); *I know* I am a food addict. Excess food is not an option (truth).

I want more control around my children (unhealthy thinking); *I know* God is taking care of them, better than I ever could (truth).

I feel hungry even after a full meal (unhealthy thinking); *I know* my food plan is nutritionally well-balanced. It is enough (truth).

I feel justified to be inconsiderate. I want to yell and scream, as was my familiar way of handling feelings (unhealthy thinking); *I know* Jesus asks me to be kind and loving. It is okay to feel angry. It is not okay to lash out and hurt people in the midst of my emotional turmoil.

I need to pray for God's guidance, accept my responsibility or contribution to the situation and make amends for my actions or attitude if they are inappropriate. Sometimes I have to "God bless" my counterpart and accept that life is not always fair. When I let go of my self-centered ego and follow Jesus, I am well. I am directed, and I find peace (truth).

> Trust in the Lord with all your heart and lean not on your own understanding; in all your ways acknowledge him, and he will make your paths straight. (Proverbs 3:5-6, *New International Version*)

Stop, Drop and Roll

When my spirit wanted to explode, there were warning signs. I'd get a gnawing in my belly. The unkind words would start to bubble up in my gut, irritating my stomach on the way to my heart. The words got ready to gush out of my mouth, when I remembered my counselor's advice, "Wait until you can respond. Out of the heart the mind speaks."

To react is an automatic response that rises out of one's emotion. Hurt people hurt people. When we feel hurt, anxious, annoyed or angry, we want to retaliate. As a food addict, I hurt myself by overeating, and I hurt others by lashing out. I yelled, complained and blamed. When I stopped overeating, I recognized my dismal attitude, accepted my brokenness and tried to correct the harm I had done. Committed to recovery, I learned new life-style skills. I learned not to react, but instead to respond in kind and loving ways. Life happens to us all: the physical maladies, the angry clerk, the inconsiderate truck driver, the too tired, sick or frustrated daycare child or the family squabble. These are all opportunities to react. *Responding in love requires the skill of self-control.*

My heart aches at times. Two examples of my growing ability to control myself come to mind. One day not long ago, being the over-protective mother that I am, I was ready to pounce on my husband for his attitude towards one of the children. Instead of attacking him with my words, I grabbed my notebook and with great vigor, wrote all the nasty things I wanted to spit at him. Later, when I settled down, I calmly and respectfully told him my thoughts. It was fruitful. He listened. In the past, he didn't hear beyond the loudness of my voice.

Communication with children holds unique challenges. I remember one day when Dan was around twelve or thirteen. Annoyed at something I had said, he strutted angrily down the hall with his nose in the air. He slammed his bedroom door and yelled, "I hate you." Initially it hurt. It hurt a lot. Before program, I would have been furious. In recovery, I waited until I could respond. It wasn't long before I realized that it was just a feeling, and feelings are not facts. Responding graciously, I said, "I see that you are upset with me. Let me know when you want to talk. I love you." Allowing my children to express their feelings helped me express mine.

One Day at a Time

Over and over again I heard, "Read page 449 in the Big Book." I read it every day as a constant reminder to let go of my anger, my defiance and my attempts to control everything and everybody. I needed to "let go and let God."

> Acceptance is the answer to *all* my problems today. When I am disturbed, it is because I find some person, place, thing, or situation—some fact of my life—unacceptable to me, and I can find no serenity until I accept that person, place, thing, or situation as being exactly the way it is supposed to be at this moment. (*Alcoholics Anonymous*, Third Edition, page 449)

Paul proclaims a similar message in his letter to the Philippians:

> ...I have learned how to be content (satisfied to the point where I am not disturbed or disquieted) in whatever state I am. (Philippians 4:11, *Amplified*).

Practicing the program was not always easy. It was "progress, not perfection." Serenity comes through never-ending acceptance and surrender, keeping our eyes on God with absolute dependence on *His* ability. "God is our refuge and strength, an ever-present help in trouble." (Psalm 46:1, *New International Version*)

The first few months were disheartening. My predisposition needed a complete overhaul. People say that it takes twenty-one days to break a habit. For me, it took eons to sever the tightly braided cords that held me captive to my compulsive and obsessive nature. One day at a time, one hour at a time, one minute at a time, I walked toward the light. Sometimes I crawled on my knees with barely enough strength to go on. It was tough. God never promised me a rose garden.

God helped me endure whatever temptations I faced. I sat on my hands some days. I went to bed some days. Talking on the telephone to other food addicts, going to a meeting or talking to my counselor revived my sprit and renewed my strength. Talking to God in casual conversations or more intimately on my knees, I did whatever I had to do to stay abstinent. It was the most important thing without exception. My old nature withered as the seeds of my new life blossomed. Celebrations, holidays and special days played havoc with my peace of mind. In God's time, the fanfare died, the commotion ended and I didn't overeat one day at a time.

> Yet this I call to mind and therefore I have hope: Because of the Lord's great love we are not consumed, for his compassions never fail. They are new every morning.... (Lamentations 3:21-23, *New International Version*)

I Think I Can...My First Baking Experience

"Happy Birthday to you...Happy Birthday to you..." Dan's fun-loving spirit and happy heart added spice to my otherwise dull day. Joe smiled contently as Dan led the way in his pre-celebration. Their shrilling voices raised the hair on the back of my neck. Neither could carry a note, but it didn't matter. Their hearts rang out loud and clear in joyful anticipation of another gala event. Feeling blessed, I thanked God for my children.

The boys and I loved to plan parties. Carl customarily groaned. He was justified to dread any "blessed" event. It was not fun for him. For years, my perfectionism gushed waves of demands on him, "Fix everything. Help me clean the entire house." It took us weeks to prepare for company. I wanted "house beautiful," and it was literally impossible to reach my absurd expectations. Try as he might to negotiate, I had a mind set in stone. Dan was turning eight and, like it or not, we were going to have a party. The date was set: October 10, 1988.

My sponsor told me to focus on the fun and games, the special things we could *do*. "Food is not the most important thing." She suggested buying a nice cake. She was dead set against my baking anything. She said, "Keep it very simple. Maybe even have friends and relatives bring food." I hesitantly agreed. It sounded reasonable, except for my groans. "Everyone expects me to have an elaborate spread. It is what I do best."

I was considering my options when Daniel broke my train of thought. "Mommy, can you make me a chocolate cake this year?" Without a moment's hesitation, I replied, "I was just thinking about that. Maybe we'll buy your cake this year." He scowled and said, "But, Mom, you *always* bake my birthday cakes." *Uh-oh, Lord, what in the world should I do?* Before program, it was my job to bake for every occasion. Any reason to celebrate, any excuse to eat some gooey, rich, delectable dessert used to be welcomed. *I have been free from compulsive overeating since the end of July, a little over two months now. Is this an accident waiting to happen?* After some serious time on my knees, I said, "I think I can do it with God's help." *Help me, Lord! My sponsor's not going to like this.*

I swallowed my fear and prepared myself for the demeaning attitude I received when I defied my sponsor's wishes. Grudgingly I dialed her number. The second she picked up the phone, I blurted out the words in one burst of energy. "I am baking on Saturday. It's Dan's birthday. He wants a homemade cake and with God's help, I can do it." I stopped to breathe, asked God for help and continued at a slower pace. "It is not an option to lick my fingers or eat any leftover anything. No batter, no frosting, not even a crumb. It is not my food."

My sponsor groaned one of those long-winded "you'll be sorry; I can't believe what I'm hearing" moans and suggested that I might want to find another sponsor. She told me directly, "If you pick up even one lick, you will *need* to find another sponsor." In retrospect, my sponsor's doubts drove my determined nature to the far ends of the earth. "I'll show her" was a thought I held onto when fighting the rising tides of temptation. Sometimes it seems as if I was wading into too-deep waters, but God kept me afloat when I was over my head.

The big event was scheduled for Saturday afternoon. Wanting help from other people, I was the first to raise my hand at the Saturday morning meeting. Openly I shared my intentions to bake my first cake. Some gasped as if I were about to commit suicide. Others encouraged me to use some simple techniques that had worked for them. "Be sure you eat your meal first" was an overwhelming "you have to." One woman offered her help: "Call me. I'll talk you through it if you want." Someone else suggested I put a band-aid on my right index finger to remind me of God's ability to heal my brokenness.

Respecting those who had gone before me, I listened. I ate my lunch, put a band-aid on my finger and commenced to bake my first cake in program. It was awkward. I never realized how many times I had cleaned the debris off my fingers by putting them in my mouth until it was no longer an option. There was a mess of paper towels covered with batter and frosting by the time I was done. That band-aid, silly as it seemed, really did work. Every time my hand came close to my mouth with a finger full of anything, I saw the band-aid and thought, "I am sick. I am a food addict. This is not my food." Chatting with God, I stayed on course.

Finally, it was time for the finishing touch. "Happy Birthday, Danny" was delicately inscribed in forest green. I stood back and admired my work. God's favor illuminated my mission. It was an awakening of sorts: A birthday cake is like an art project. I had created a masterpiece and a labor of love, no less. Considering the substance was not edible, for me anyway, it was like knitting a sweater or building a dollhouse. I was jubilant. From that moment on, I have never had a problem baking or distributing pastries at a party. My spirit soared. *Praise the Lord: "I can do everything with the help of Christ who gives me the strength I need."* (Philippians 4:13, *New Living*)

Pleased as punch, I reveled in my accomplishment. Immediately I called my sponsor to proclaim the good news, "I did it and it's beautiful." My enthusiasm gushed. I was anxious to share my art project awakening, but her dead silence stunned me. I asked, "Are you there?" On the other end of the line, I was attacked by her snide interrogation, "You mean you didn't take even one lick? That's hard to believe." Temporarily deflated by her accusations, I said to myself, "There is no pleasing this woman." *Lord, You know I am telling the truth. You were there.* I "God blessed her" and shrugged my shoulders one more time.

My counselor often encouraged me by saying, "Take what you want and leave the rest. You need to go to the waterholes that fill you." I telephoned the women from the meeting who had encouraged me earlier that day. I thanked them for their help and grabbed the opportunity to share my newfound revelation: "Baking is like creating an art project. I made a beautiful masterpiece today." They marveled at my message and considered it "food for thought" in the future. I heard many testimonies of others who gained wisdom and strength from my experience.

> Two people can accomplish more than twice as much as one; they get a better return for their labor. If one person falls, the other can reach out and help. But people who are alone when they fall are in real trouble.... Three are even better, for a triple-braided cord is not easily broken. (Ecclesiastes 4:9-12, *New Living Translation*)

As I drifted off to sleep that night, peace and joy filled my soul. The program is people helping people with dependence and trust in God's ability. *The Third Step Prayer worked again. Continue to use me, Lord Jesus, if it is Your will.*

I Think I Can...My First Halloween

"Trick or Treat? Smell my feet. Give me something good to eat." The children's jovial voices chimed in unison.

Halloween was Carl's favorite holiday. He happily volunteered to chaperone the children throughout the neighborhood. My assignment was to distribute the candy to the trick-or-treaters. The task may sound easy, but maybe not.

Alone, with my favorite food in the whole wide world, I waited for the doorbell to ring. *It's Halloween and everyone eats candy on Halloween. Maybe I could have just one piece. I'll pick my favorite treat. I'll be fine. Just one piece won't hurt. Who would know? What difference would it make? Lord, what should I do?*

I remembered my commitment. My food is my food and everything else is not my food. I picked up the telephone. I was not alone. My friend on the other end of the line was contemplating her options, too. She said what I was thinking, "Maybe just one piece?" We talked about the trials and tribulations of being food addicts and wallowed in self-pity for a while. We were angry that we could not enjoy Halloween. In time, we remembered that it had been years since we actually enjoyed the food fests that accompanied the holiday, and we laughed at our crazy thinking. We both agreed that one bite is a binge for a food addict. It was not an option to overeat, even on Halloween. I hung up the telephone and thanked God for helping me fight the incredible temptations of the holiday. With renewed strength, I dialed other compulsive overeaters.

Carl, Dan and Joe returned with their hauls. My husband was a peach. He volunteered to take full responsibility of the boys' treats. It was tough for me to let go of my need to control everything, but I knew in the pit of my being that it was the right thing to do. He distributed the candy to the boys each day, giving them one or two pieces at a time.

Out of the goodness of his heart, Carl hid the remaining goodies just in case I got tempted. For the first time in my life, I understood the expression, "Out of sight, out of mind." Wow, huh? I was surprised and impressed. God deserved the credit. I was getting better at surrendering my will and my life over to His care each day, slowly and with each baby step.

I Think I Can...My First Wedding Reception

The wedding was beautiful. It was a match made in heaven. On the way to the reception, I drifted off to "la-la land" and imagined being like everyone else. *If I were normal, this could be fun. I would be eating, drinking and dancing*. Carl's nudge woke me up. He was looking for directions. I told him the exit we needed to take and then I asked, "Do you ever wish we were normal?" He rolled his eyes as if to say, "Don't ask such a stupid question." He kept silent. I thought about page 449 in the Big Book. You need to accept life on life's term. "Acceptance is the answer to all my problems today." *Okay, I accept that I am a food addict, and Carl is an alcoholic. Carl cannot drink alcohol. I cannot overeat. Maybe we can help each other.*

I knew what to expect. I had called the restaurant and discussed my dietary restrictions as a food addict weeks before the big day. For safety's sake, I restated my intentions to my husband. "Carl, I can eat the chicken, the red bliss potatoes, the cooked vegetable and a dry salad. I brought my salad dressing. I know you love me and want me to be happy. I need to remember that extra food is not the answer anymore. Please do not suggest *any* other foods. This is my plan." My voice elevated with each line. *Lord, help me to stay abstinent today.* Somewhat intimidated by my spiteful spirit, he nodded his head indicating that he understood my instructions.

Carl and I had history. My dear husband got the brunt of my anger. He witnessed baffled and confused moments of utter dismay when my determined nature would dissolve midstream. Being far too proud to tell him I had blown another great plan, I'd often sneak eat. He hadn't a clue. Trying to be helpful, he would say some innocent remark in hopes of supporting "the plan." The poor man would get slapped in the face with my sneer. My nasty disposition would knock him off his feet, "Leave me alone. I'll eat what I want. *You* don't know what it's like to be a food addict."

Carl had his own cross to bear. This was his first wedding without alcohol and it was open bar. Our anxiety levels rose as we approached the magnificent resort. Carl couldn't drink, and I couldn't overeat.

What a team! Almost traumatized with fearful anticipation, we agreed that a cup of coffee might be nice. The car veered off course, and we landed at the local coffee shop. We sat, almost paralyzed, and collected our thoughts.

The detour held no serious repercussions. We arrived at the reception site before the newlyweds, which was proper etiquette. Waiters and waitresses were milling around the exquisite resort offering fabulous hors d'oeuvres. Carl seemed to forget about drinking. He basked in the consumption of the culinary delights, delectable scallops wrapped in bacon, "giant jumbo, super-sized shrimp" (his words) and stuffed mushrooms. I took mine for him. It was our routine. If I couldn't eat it, I forced my share on him. This time, he didn't mind.

It seemed like hours later when the bride and groom entered the scene. They were introduced as Mr. and Mrs. for the first time. My stomach was growling. My patience was wearing thin. I was enviously watching the cordial little gatherings of family and friends. Everyone looked happy and content to mingle. *Of course, they were happy; they were stuffing themselves with all that food.*

Finally, in God's sweet time, we were invited to find our seats in the Camelot Room. The hostess told us that it was time for the meal. People munched on the fresh baked rolls still warm from the oven. Many raved over "the exquisite pecan twirls." Impatiently I waited and waited some more. Carl could see the tension mounting. The poor man looked scared. I felt like a simmering pot of water getting ready to boil. He tried to calm me, "Relax, it will be okay." He had noticed a waitress in the distance. "They are serving the salads now." Smiling ever so slightly, I took another sip of my water.

When the waitress placed a puny plate of greens in front of me, my eyes welled up. I whispered in anguish, "This is a garnish, not a salad." Carl pushed his over to me, trying desperately to console me, and said, "Baby, you can have mine." I held back my tears and uttered indignantly, "Thank you." After what seemed like forever, the main meal was served. I sighed a "thank-you, God" and polished-off the reasonable portion of chicken, three red bliss potatoes and the four green beans that were "the cooked vegetable." I tried, with all my might, to say, "It's okay. Some meals are not ideal. You won't die." I found solace in remembering that my next meal was a normal dinner, which was prepared and waiting at home for whenever we returned. I had followed my plan to the best of my ability. The coffee was served and the dancing began.

We stepped onto the dance floor and shuffled our feet through one song. Without alcohol, Carl was not inclined to be in any spotlight. It was okay with me. I liked the shelter of his wing. We sat and watched the others and enjoyed some casual chitchat.

It was time to cut the wedding cake. It was a scrumptious-looking carrot cake with cream cheese frosting. We watched the bride and groom's lovely interchange. My mind started roaming into dreamland. *Maybe I could have a small piece. I was so "good" at lunch. Who would know?* I was in trouble. I considered my commitment to my sponsor and tried to rationalize having one piece. *My vegetables were skimpy at lunch; this cake is made with carrots. I can do this.* I took my piece. Carl looked at me. Nervously he said, "Are you bringing some cake home for the boys?" *Lord, help me.* I nodded my head and wrapped it in my napkin. *Okay, Lord, I won't eat it right now.*

I placed it ever so gently next to my purse. Relishing the thought of its indescribably delicious taste, I eyed it for the rest of the day. I brought it home and placed it on the counter. *Lord, what should I do? God's still small voice said, "Not for today."* Begrudgingly I said, "Okay, I won't eat it today." I threw it in the freezer and wondered if I would be strong enough to resist the temptation tomorrow. *Tomorrow is not here. Just for today, I have a plan.* The next day came. On my knees I asked, "Lord, should I have that cake today?" The answer was the same, "not today, tomorrow you can ask again."

All of my favorites were stashed in the freezer for "tomorrow." Candy, cookies and special treats, peanut butter cups, chocolate chip cookies, white chocolate were all waiting in the freezer. Self-destruction lurked in the freezer. *Lord, help me. Just for today, I will follow my plan. Tomorrow I'll ask again.* In time, months later, I stopped collecting forbidden foods in the freezer. I gained a sure foundation and rejoiced in the truth that sugar and flour are poison for a food addict. I recoil from these "drugs" as one would from a hot flame, just one day at a time.

> So don't worry about tomorrow, for tomorrow will bring its own worries. Today's trouble is enough for today. (Matthew 6:34, *New Living Translation*)

I Think I Can...My First Thanksgiving

"We gather together to ask the Lord's blessing." *Thanksgiving* is *God's blessings?* Thanksgiving is a day of food with wonderful, fancy, mouth-watering baked goods and an elaborate turkey dinner with all the trimmings, stuffing, gravies, mashed potatoes and fancy vegetable casseroles. Life, as I had known it, was over.

I committed my food to my sponsor: "turkey, vegetables without sugar or flour, mashed potatoes and a salad. I'll bring my salad dressing." *What am I going to do today? I wish I could say that I was sick. I want to stay home. I hate this, no breads, no desserts, no gravy, no stuffing, no "good" stuff. Okay, Lord, I need You to do this for me today. I am sick. I have the disease of food addiction.*

My food is my food. Everything else is not my food, even on Thanksgiving. Help me, Lord.

The relatives arrived. I smiled and acted as if it was great to be together for the holiday. The truth: I was miserable. I wanted to disown my food addiction. Angrily I watched like an outsider. People were sampling the new concoctions and praising the chefs for their creative contributions. The old standbys called my name: the butterscotch pie, the date nut bread, the crispy edge of the stuffing dipped in the turkey grease, all the tried and true favorites for me. Drooling on the inside, I must have looked downright disheartened. My well-meaning relatives said, "Lighten up. Live a little for one day." Too many times, I heard, "Pam, you have done so well. Nobody diets on Thanksgiving. Just go back on your diet tomorrow." Quietly I murmured, "Thanks, but no thanks." I tried to be polite, but I wanted to scream, "I CANNOT OVEREAT TODAY. I am sick. I have a disease. LEAVE ME ALONE." I wanted to go home. I wanted to run. I wanted to escape. I wanted to jump over some hurdle onto safe ground. *Please help me, Lord.*

In my family, Thanksgiving was a day to excuse overeating. I did it for years. It was another tradition. My family didn't diet on any holiday: Thanksgiving, Christmas or on any special occasion. I vowed that this year was different. I made a solemn promise to stay abstinent and with the help of God, I stayed true to my plan, but it was a very l-o-n-g day. I paced in circles, tried to do some small talk, took trips to the bathroom where I fell to my knees in quiet desperation and waited for the day to end.

Around 7 P.M., in preparation to leave, people gathered their portions of the leftovers, which was another tradition in my family. For the first time in my life, we said, "good night" and went home empty-handed with no food to enjoy for the rest of the day in the comfort of my own home, as was my usual after-the-holiday ritual. I was sad and tired. I said a half-hearted "thank you" to God, and I went to bed emotionally exhausted.

Many days, weeks and months passed after those first few challenging events, and different days presented unique obstacles, but I stayed true to my plan. Was it easy? No way. Was it possible? With God's help, all things are possible. I learned to accept life on life's terms. When I thought about food or some person, place, thing or situation that disturbed my peace of mind, I made a phone call. I attended a meeting or I did some form of love and service. I focused my attention on productive, helpful activities. I stopped fighting and I surrendered each new day. Thy will, not mine, be done.

Who Is Your God?

"Pam, have you been sick? You look awful." My sick head smiled at the remarks of some family members and close friends who voiced their concerns about my too thin body. When they gasped at my appearance, I somehow felt successful, as if I had reached some unspeakable ideal.

One day I reluctantly asked my sponsor how much she thought I should weigh. She told me about her guidelines: "In order to stop the weight games, I follow the well-known rule of thumb, which is 100 lbs. for the first five feet and add 5 pounds for each inch after that." We calculated my targeted goal. I am five foot seven inches tall. Therefore, my goal weight is 135 lbs. Allowing a ten-pound range, I could weigh anywhere between 125 lbs. and 135 lbs. My doctor agreed with this calculation, but I was doubtful. I thought 118 lbs. sounded more appealing or maybe even 110 lbs.

My sponsor told me to weigh-in on the first day of each month. She said, "Focus your attention on recovery, not on the numbers you see on the scale." She added, "As you follow your food plan each new day, trust that you will maintain a thin body. Practice the slogan, 'Let go and let God.'"

Fear of falling back into my old habits of overeating or not eating enough kept me chained tightly to my witness of success, the number on the scale. That metal monster sat on my bathroom floor, and I did not ignore it. I reported my weight once a month, *but* I weighed myself more often. Sometimes I weighed in once a week, sometimes on the first and the fifteenth of the month, sometimes every day. Bottom line: *the scale ruled me.* It affected my attitude about myself; when I was 128 lbs. or less, I felt successful and happy. Nothing above 128 lbs. was okay. Even though my food plan had not changed, I felt like a "bad girl." My disposition often changed in the blink of an eye. I went from happy and optimistic to gloom and doom. Being an extremist, I imagined myself fat overnight if I didn't *do* something different immediately. In time, my program friends and my experience taught me that my weight would fluctuate. It is natural, normal, and okay.

Years into program, an eating disorder specialist told me that she threw her scale away. I looked at her in awe and said, "I could never do that." She smiled and asked, "Are you trusting God or are you controlling your weight?" I explained that it is the action of my hand that feeds me. She said, "I know if I start eating more than my body needs that the fit of my clothes will tell me to eat less food."

I have not thrown my scale away, but I have let the "boogie man" sit there, unnoticed, for months at a time. Occasionally I do check in, just to see, and it feels like the right thing for me to do at this stage in my life, because I know the tricks I played in the past. I can be conniving: I avoid weighing in so I can get thinner. *If I see that I weigh less than 125 lbs., I'll have to add food.* On the other hand, I ignore the scale when my clothes are feeling snug, because I know I should eliminate some food from my plan. *If I see that I am over 135 lbs., then I'll have to cut something out and I don't want to do that.*

My conclusion: if I am not willing to change anything, it is fruitless to weigh myself. It serves only as a means to beat myself up.

Touchdown

For a while, I enjoyed parading around in the latest fashions. I wore cute little ditties bought "off the rack" in popular sizes, and I soaked in all the compliments. I felt like a movie star. Well-intentioned family and friends encouraged me to let down my guard, especially on the holidays. They said, "A little treat won't hurt you." Or "Now that you're thin, you certainly don't need to diet anymore." They didn't understand the disease of food addiction. It was okay. It was hard for me to accept the fact that I was done losing weight. I had a fat head and no matter how thin I got, I still envisioned myself as heavy. Even today, when I catch a glimpse of my reflection in a mirror or in a storefront window, I am surprised that the woman looking back at me is thin.

Still thinking thinner would be better; my new venture (obsession) became the act of physical fitness. It became my new preoccupation: where, when and how to get physically fit. I need to tell you that it was not for medical reasons, but for sheer vanity. My thin body was pear shaped or people might say that I was "bottom heavy," and my legs were flabby. I felt that these deficits could be fixed with the right exercises. Therefore, I joined health clubs, bought exercise equipment and dreamed of the day when I would have the perfect body.

One day I sought help with my priorities. God blessed me with an insight. I heard, "Stop working on your body. Beauty is only skin deep." I knew it was wise to incorporate exercise in my life, but it was also wise to spend time with God, and I wanted to help other people in the program. I needed to make some choices. After some *serious* consideration, I said, "Okay, Lord. What should I do?"

Walking satisfied my physical needs, and it enhanced my spirit. Monday through Friday, I take a two-mile walk early in the morning, right after my prayer and meditation time with God. When I walk, I feel refreshed and alive. It is the best of both worlds. The physical and spiritual spheres meet on the road to a better life.

When I finally succumbed to the idea that thinner is not better, I embarked on the most difficult phase of recovery, which is maintenance. It was time to share my story. "I am not only on a diet with an exercise regime. I am in a program to learn how to live."

> Physical exercise has some value, but spiritual exercise is much more important, for it promises a reward in both this life and the next. (1 Timothy 4:8, *New Living Translation*)

Denial is Not Just a River in Egypt

"Food secrets? Do I have any food secrets?" My sponsor's inquiry startled me. *Oh no, I'm in big trouble. Help me, Lord.* I was caught with my hand in the cookie jar. My conniving, defiant nature was exposed. I grabbed the dictionary, hoping for a way out. I read that a secret is something hidden or concealed. An implied truth is a secret. It is dishonest and establishes guilt by omission.

When I was overly anxious, I gave myself permission to overeat abstinent food. I would often make an excuse to eat at a wonderful restaurant. Buffets served me well. If I couldn't get my husband to take me out to dinner, I would opt for plan two. I slyly committed my food. I would say, "I'm barbecuing steak tonight with baked potatoes, 1 cup of broccoli, 2 cups of salad, 1 T. salad dressing and a fruit." I had added a fruit for dinner when I reached my goal weight. In lieu of my reasonably weighed and measured portions, I gnawed the meat off a delicious T-bone steak, which weighed at least a pound, probably more. My potato was gigantic; I would travel from market to market to find the biggest, most beautiful potato in town. Moreover, my piece of fruit was huge. After I ate one of these meals, I would say to myself, "That was not a great idea, but I was not that "bad." I only had ONE steak, ONE potato and ONE piece of fruit. My vegetables and salad were measured. If I were overeating, it would have been a lot worse. At least the meal ended."

I also played with other protein choices, "I'm cooking a Cornish hen for dinner tonight, and I'll have xyz." I intentionally refrained from committing my portion size once again. I ate the whole hen (probably 1o-12 oz.), and I sucked every edible ounce of meat off those bones (including skin, fat and cartilage, no less). Only a pile of twigs (the empty bones) remained. It was a sad, unreasonable choice. I was guilty once again.

Another consistent justification/rationalization: I remember measuring my food and even though the scale said, "6.2 oz." instead of "6.0" or "4.3 oz." instead of "4.0," I decided that it was close enough, and I ate the whole portion. Nutritionally, it didn't make much of a difference, but it was still not okay. This is a program of honesty.

All these incidents and more were certainly occasions when I overate. Denial is not just a river in Egypt. It's the little exceptions (secrets) that pile up to cause resentments, which grow and eventually could become a reason to binge.

I had food secrets. I had many food secrets. My journal held the truth and God knew. *Lord, help me. I want to be well. My food plan is enough.* I got honest, scrupulously honest, and I confessed every indiscretion. Finally, I understood how to be abstinent. I was honest, open and willing. I even discussed restaurants, buffets and special celebrations in detail. My sponsor and I designed a plan each day, and I did what I planned. For the first time I understood freedom. I was happy to be in recovery. It was simple, satisfying and without guilt.

> The program of action, though entirely sensible, was pretty drastic. It meant I would have to throw several lifelong conceptions out of the window. That was not easy. But the moment I made up my mind to go through with the process, I had the curious feeling that my alcoholic [addictive] condition was relieved, as in fact it proved to be. (*Alcoholics Anonymous,* Third Edition, page 42)

New Light

The sun was shining, the birds were singing, and I was ready for a brand new day. I tied my sneakers, strapped my radio to my belt and headed outside for my morning walk. I moved the dial of the radio hoping to find something to ponder during my half-hour jaunt. News, weather, sports, rap, loud music, *isn't there anything interesting out there in the world?* I continued my search and stopped in my tracks when I heard a woman's raspy voice boldly proclaim, "Jesus can heal the brokenhearted. When Jesus heals, the lame walk and the blind see!" It was Joyce Meyer, a powerful television and radio minister. Immediately, she touched the core of my being with her inspiring testimony. I heard about Jesus. Through the Word of God, her life had changed.

As soon as I walked into the house, I grabbed my Bible. I searched for the Scripture Joyce had talked about. It was Isaiah 61. She had quoted from *The Amplified Bible,* which was far different from my *King James Version.* My *King James Version* was written in words that were harder for me to understand, but the message remained clear. For easier interpretation, this reference comes from the *New Living Translation:*

> The Spirit of the Sovereign Lord is upon me, because the Lord has appointed me to bring good news to the poor. He has sent me to comfort the brokenhearted and to announce that captives will be released and prisoners will be freed. He has sent me to tell those who mourn that the time of the Lord's favor has come... he will give beauty for ashes, joy instead of mourning, praise instead of despair...
>
> They will rebuild the ancient ruins, repairing cities long ago destroyed. They will revive them, though they have been empty for many generations... Instead of shame and dishonor, you will inherit a double portion of prosperity and everlasting joy. (Isaiah 61:1-7, *New Living Translation*)

My mind's eye saw that God had "released" me and other people who were once actively addicted to food. We had been held "captive" to the disease. I saw that joy does come when we strive to rebuild our lives, and that we will be blessed more than we could have ever imagined, if we follow the teaching of Jesus.

Immediately I knew that God had bigger plans for my life. At this point in my recovery, I was relatively happy. I thought at the time that my life was as good as it could be. I was abstinent and getting better physically and emotionally through the help of the Twelve Steps. Spiritually, I was certainly dependent on God, but new light dawned this day. It was another spiritual awakening of sorts: The Big Book had been my "Bible;" it had brought me to this stage of my recovery, but God wanted more for me.

> Blessed are those who hunger and thirst for righteousness, for they will be filled. (Matthew 5:6, *New International Version*)

I became a dedicated fan of Joyce Meyer overnight. I was a baby in the Lord, but my understanding and application of Biblical principles grew steadily as I absorbed the teaching of her program *Life in the Word* each new day.

Open my eyes to see wonderful things in your Word. I am but a pilgrim here on earth: how I need a map—and your commands are my chart and guide. I long for your instructions more than I can tell. (Psalm 119:18-20, *The Living Bible*)

Higher Ground

When I was a child, I talked like a child, I thought like a child, I reasoned like a child. When I became a man, I put childish ways behind me. (1 Corinthians 13:11, *New International Version*)

As children, we set out to explore new territory. Unknowingly we engage in dangerous activities. We climb on furniture, run when we should walk, hide in public places and the like. We test the waters and discover the boundaries of our safety zones. When a caring adult witnesses a potentially harmful situation, he or she automatically warns children of hazards and declares, "Danger! Chairs are for sitting." Or "We walk in the house." If a child falls, he learns that the adult was trying to protect him; it hurts when you fall. In time, children grow into self-nurturing, independent adults.

A sponsor is like the good parent or a personal trainer. A sponsor is someone who suggests certain guidelines, methods and philosophies to induce positive lifestyle changes. In the program, whining occurs from time to time.

Mistakes are inevitable. People need appropriate redirection. It is all part of the process.

My sponsor's commitment to abstinence was impressive. She went to any length to stay abstinent. She was sure-footed in her understanding of the 12-step program. I needed a firm hand, although I acted like a baby when she suggested I get down off "that dangerous chair." Beyond my immaturity, we had one major difference in opinion. She believed in a higher power, the God of her understanding, which appeared to be the group or the program in general. I had a more defined God, the God of the Bible. Frustration and confusion arose periodically. God would tell me one thing, and she would tell me another. She said, "You're a baby. After a year, you can make your own decisions."

For months, I fought the temptation to say, "I'm outta here." Feeling suffocated by her control, I often wondered if she was the right sponsor for me. Each time I got on my knees to pray about it, I heard, "Be patient. Your sponsor can teach you discipline and self-control."

> Fools think they need no advice, but the wise listen to others. (Proverbs 12:15, *New Living Translation*)

A Leap of Faith

When I succumbed to her teaching technique and acknowledged that I had changed by her persistent efforts, I thanked her. Then one day God said, "*Now* you can fly." I knew in my heart that it was time to depend on Him.

> I will instruct you and teach you in the way you should go; I will counsel you and watch over you" [says the Lord.] (Psalm 32:8, *New International Version*)

My disciplines were in place, I had self-control, and I knew that abstinence was the most important thing without exception. It was not an option to overeat no matter what was happening in my circumstances or how I felt. I was ready to grow up.

One exceptionally bright and sunny day in December, I dialed the number of my sponsor for the last time as her underling. Graciously, with respect and love, I shared what the Lord had said to me. It didn't matter whether she understood it or not. I was free to soar for Him now. It was almost an angelic, out-of-body experience. My feet barely touching the ground, I said to the Lord, "Here I am. I am ready to do Your will."

> But those who hope in the Lord will renew their strength. They will soar on wings like eagles; they

will run and not grow weary, they will walk and not be faint. (Isaiah 40:31, *New International Version*)

The 12-step program taught me that I was not an island. Accountability is crucial to ongoing recovery. Another long-term abstinent member of the program volunteered to listen to my food each day. Enthusiastically, she said, "We can help each other." It was a different connection. My new sponsor believed in Jesus. It was easy to verbalize our opinions in kind and loving suggestions, possibilities or helpful hints. We bounced ideas back and forth and depended on God as the ultimate authority. We were sisters in the Lord, prayer partners and best friends.

Love is patient, love is kind. It does not envy, it does not boast, it is not proud. It is not rude, it is not self-seeking, it is not easily angered, it keeps no record of wrongs. Love does not delight in evil but rejoices with the truth. It always protects, always trusts, always hopes, always perseveres. Love never fails.... (1 Corinthians 13:4-8, *New International Version*)

Sweet Tooth

My co-sponsor and I were equal partners with the same goals of physical, emotional and spiritual health. We agreed that honesty, accountability and listening to God's instructions were pivotal to our success.

Abstinence was our first topic of conversation. She had gotten her food plan from a treatment center years before our encounter. Up to this point, I was eating the standard food plan, three meals a day with nothing in between, except black coffee, tea or water. We compared the two plans. My protein portions at lunch and dinner were 4 oz. (or ½ cup). She had 3 oz. (or l/3 cup), and at lunch she had a grain instead of a fruit. I groaned for a minute until she said, "I eat a snack before bed." I smiled. It was breakfast again and time for another oatmeal, yogurt and fruit. She said, "It is a metabolic adjustment." That sounded inviting to me and well balanced nutritionally.

She continued, "I measure my food on a digital scale. My plastic cups were warped from my stuffing every last morsel into them." I could relate to that. I would squish down the food. When I took my hand off the top, the food would bounce back. It was my food, but I occasionally wondered if it was really honest. *Did other people push the limits like me?* I bought a digital scale and started my new food plan the next day.

Breakfast: l oz. (measured dry) oatmeal or oat bran, 8 oz. plain yogurt and a fruit (Note: the cereal was cooked in ¾ cup of water.)

Lunch: 3 oz. protein, 6 oz. cooked vegetables, 8 oz. salad, 1 tablespoon salad dressing and one grain—one potato or 4 oz. rice or two plain rice cakes.

Dinner: lunch again.

Metabolic: breakfast again.

As we exchanged our bottom lines of abstinence, she said, "I don't eat sugar, flour or caffeine." I took a deep breath and groaned, "No coffee?" She told me that caffeine is another addictive drug. We discussed it rationally and concluded that we could have different bottom lines. I said, "If God leads me to stop drinking coffee, then I will stop drinking coffee."

She confessed that she ate some artificially sweetened foods. My ears perked up. In a matter of minutes, I headed for the door. *If it worked for her, it could work for me.* I briefly raced the idea of adding artificially sweetened foods by God, but I don't remember stopping long enough to hear his response. I ran to the grocery store and bought all those yummy, artificially sweetened nonfat yogurts that I loved and diet soda by the gallons. Yahoo! I was happy, four meals a day, my caffeine hits and now artificially sweetened options. Life was sweet.

There's No Place Like Home

Time passed quickly. It seemed like days and I was celebrating five years of abstinence. It was a miracle, a gift from God. Participating in many in-depth studies of the Twelve Steps, I shared my growing faith. Jesus continued to heal my broken heart, mind and body. At some meetings, people frowned at my enthusiasm for God. Feeling discouraged and persecuted, I got thirsty for more teaching and for more like-minded people in my life. *Lord, help me to know and do Your will.* Instinctively, I started praying for a church home.

This was not the first time that I had investigated the possibilities. The boys and I had visited different churches from time to time through the years, but we never found a place that kept our attention for very long. In my opinion, most church services were boring. It had been my experience that services with rote prayers and rituals from pre-written manuscripts lacked thought and feeling. I wanted and needed more. I didn't know what the "more" looked like because I had never found "it."

In a matter of weeks, God answered my prayer. Dan was fifteen; he had a friend whose family actively attended a non-denominational Christ-centered church in a nearby town. One day Dan was invited to attend. I think it was a bribe of some sort. His friend appeared a tad rebellious, but was obliged to go to church with his parents and a younger brother. He may have said, "Do you want to come to church with us? We can do something fun after the service." Apprehensively Dan asked, "What do you think, Mom, should I go?" I thought it was a great idea. Dan went and I tagged along.

It was a big church. I felt lost amongst the people, but I heard the message of hope loud and clear. "Jesus is alive" rang from beam to beam. The church was a trek from our home, but I continued to attend regular services, until one treacherous day. It was midwinter and the snow-covered streets were almost impassable. Trying to maneuver on the slick roads, I felt God say, "It is dangerous driving today. It is okay to go to church in the town where you live. I will be there, too."

> ...where two or three come together in my name, there I am with them. (Matthew 18:20, *New International Version*)

I looked up towards the sky as if God were sitting on a cloud, and asked, "Where should I go?" The boys and I had already investigated most of the local churches, including the Catholic, the Congregational and the Episcopal. I suddenly remembered "the little church on the hill." I drove into the parking lot of Faith Baptist Church. I was "home" the minute I walked into the sanctuary.

It was a quaint little church with a handful of people at the time. The gospel was presented through nontraditional services, drama and special music. It was odd to me at first. There were guitars, drums and people clapping and having fun in church. In the blink of an eye, I joined the many who easily expressed their love for the Lord. I felt united in spirit and in truth. My needs were met. I was welcomed and loved. *Home at last, home at last. Thank God, I'm home at last.* My childlike faith grew rapidly as I became involved in Bible studies and various small group ministries.

My excitement overflowed into my home life. In a matter of a few short weeks, my boys were dropping in at various church functions to see for themselves what I was experiencing. Gradually God called them. I had waited and continued to pray for them each step along the way. Eventually they became active members of the church. *Praise the Lord.* My husband, on the other hand, came occasionally and enjoyed the services and some of the outreach events. As of this writing, he still has not been "called" to join us on a regular basis. I wait in continual prayer.

Rise and Shine

> Make every effort to add to your faith goodness; and to goodness, knowledge; and to knowledge, self-control; and to self-control, perseverance; and to perseverance, godliness; and to godliness, brotherly kindness; and to brotherly kindness, love. For if you possess these qualities in increasing measure, they will keep you from being ineffective and unproductive in your knowledge of our Lord Jesus Christ. (2 Peter 1:5-8, *New International Version*)

The church's basic philosophy is designed around Willow Creek Community Church, South Barrington, Illinois. People are taught the Biblical principles of living well, loving deeply and serving the Lord according to their passions and abilities. If there is a need in the church, it is essential that the person filling the position had been called by God to do the job. Teachers are people who are called by God to teach, not just a warm body filling a need. It was the same with every job in the church. Hostesses are people with the gift of hospitality, deacons have the gift of mercy and pastors have the gift of evangelism and shepherding.

> We have different gifts, according to the grace given us. If a man's gift is prophesying, let him

use it in proportion to his faith. If it is serving, let him serve; if it is teaching, let him teach; if it is encouraging, let him encourage; if it is contributing to the needs of others, let him give generously; if it is leadership, let him govern diligently; if it is showing mercy, let him do it cheerfully. (Romans 12:6-8, *New International Version*)

The mission of my church is to edify the body of believers and glorify God. With that in mind, Pastor Doug led a teaching seminar called Networking. He hoped to fit people into their passions, not just at church, but also in every phase of life. Enthusiastically I grabbed the opportunity to find my place and my purpose.

Evaluating my heartfelt desires, as well as my unique talents and abilities, brought me to the conclusion that I was naturally endowed with faith, mercy, teaching and shepherding.

At home and in my career as a Christian daycare provider, I was "in my passion." I taught children at an early age how to trust and believe in God's awesome ability and unfailing love. My other passion was equally endearing. I longed to touch the hearts of people with addictions. I wanted to teach them about Jesus, bridging the gap between Twelve-Step programs and Christianity. *How could I teach other people with addictions about Jesus?* Praying diligently, I sought a solution. My answer came when I spotted *The Twelve Steps for Christians* by RPI at a local bookstore.

> *The Twelve Steps for Christians*, Revised Edition is a powerful resource for merging the practical wisdom of the Twelve Steps with the spiritual truths of the Bible. This combination of recovery and spirituality offers Christians an effective way to work a traditional Twelve-Step program and name Jesus Christ as their Higher Power. (Friends in Recovery, *The Twelve Steps for Christians*, RPI Publishing, back cover)

Shortly thereafter, *The Twelve Steps for Christians* Support Group was birthed at Faith Baptist Church in Auburn, MA. It has run nonstop since the year 1996. I thank the Lord each time I see another soul touched by the light of God's amazing grace. God began a good work in me, and He will be faithful to complete it. (See Philippians 1:6.)

It was my first introduction to The Serenity Prayer in its entirety:

> God, grant me the serenity to accept the things I cannot change, the courage to change the things I can, and the wisdom to know the difference. Living one day at a time, enjoying one moment at a time, accepting hardship as a pathway to peace; taking, as Jesus did, this sinful world as it is, not as I would have it; trusting that You will make all

things right if I surrender to your will; so that I may be reasonably happy in this life and supremely happy with You forever in the next. Amen. (by Reinhold Niebuhr)

Good to the Last Drop

The Twelve Steps for Christians Support Group addressed life's issues. There were people from all walks of life, including food addicts, alcoholics, co-dependents, plus adult children of alcoholics, people working on fears, depression or whatever separated them from God. It was fruitful, and we multiplied.

One summer day, I was at a tag sale and I happened to pick up an interesting book called *The All New Free to be Thin* by Neva Coyle and Marie Chapian. It was a Biblically-based study for people with food issues. Stimulated by new insights, I gathered the troops, so to speak, and led a teaching for thirteen weeks as outlined in the *Lifestyle Plan*, which was a personal journal written to accompany the textbook. Members from the church and fellow food addicts joined me in this venture. The food addicts ignored the food plan. It was a nutritionally balanced diet for a *normal* eater. The people from the church, who were looking for self-control and behavior modification, followed the food plan suggested.

God blessed many people with increased understanding. Personally, I was convicted of my coffee and artificial sweetener addiction. They were my last "drugs," my last obsessions. I came to realize that I held onto them in lieu of appearing a perfectionist or extremist. *People already think my food plan is extreme and fanatically strict. Coffee and artificial sweeteners are normal foods for a dieter. I want to appear normal.* God gently assured me that I was not "normal." Lovingly I heard, "I have called you to higher ground." He asked me to lay these things at His feet. I let go of what other people thought of me and my food plan, and I listened.

I need to tell you a secret. *I loved my coffee.* It was my shot in the arm when I needed a boost. I drank it twenty-four hours a day, seven days a week, when I began my stretch of back-to-back abstinence in 1988. Through the years, though, I heard people share that caffeine was a drug to be avoided. It created unclear thinking, and it was addicting. I chose to ignore those comments. *Lord, I love my coffee, and I have already sacrificed so much. I can keep it; right, Lord?* The answer was obvious.

Eventually I weaned down to three cups a day, then two, then one, though it was one *enormous* cup. My husband often tells the story of my "soup bowl" of coffee. It was *one* cup. That was the best I could do for a very long time.

Decaffeinated coffee worked for a short span, but I soon played games to mask my denial. I wanted my caffeine hit. I would make it triple strength and let the first few splashes fall directly into my cup or I would order a large cup from the best coffee shops knowing that their decaffeinated coffee was more potent than other establishments. When I started the *Free to be Thin* program, I was resigned to one cup of decaffeinated coffee a day. I held onto it with both hands, until I read Romans, Chapter 12.

> And so, dear brother and sisters, I plead with you to give your bodies to God. Let them be a living and holy sacrifice—the kind he will accept. When you think of what he has done for you, is this too much to ask? Don't copy the behavior and customs of this world, but let God transform you into a new person by changing the way you think. Then you will know what God wants you to do, and you will know how good and pleasing and perfect his will really is. (Romans l2:l-2, *New Living Translation*)

I offered everything to God. I surrendered my coffee and at the same time, I said "good-bye" to my artificially sweetened yogurts and my occasional diet sodas. I learned to love pure, natural water and plain yogurt. I considered them treasures and close to the heart of God's natural state of creation.

> Everything is permissible—but not everything is beneficial... (1 Corinthians 10:23, New International Version)

Making the decision to treat food as a prescription drug, I eat only foods that nourish my body. Never have I felt so free and so alive. Willingness is a gift from heaven.

> So if the Son sets you free, you will indeed be free. (John 8:36, *New Living Translation*)

The Good Fight

All battles belong to the Lord. In Biblical times, Jehoshaphat was at war. Overwhelmed with approaching armies, he cried out to God.

> O our God, won't you stop them? We are powerless against this mighty army that is about to attack us. We do not know what to do, but we are looking to you for help. (2 Chronicles 20:12, *New Living Translation*)

I can certainly relate. *Lord, won't you take this food addiction from me? I am powerless over all the temptations in the world. I cannot do this alone. Help me, Lord Jesus.*

> ...This is what the Lord says: Do not be afraid! Don't be discouraged by this mighty army, for the

battle is not yours, but God's. Tomorrow, march out against them...you will not even need to fight. Take your positions; then stand still and watch the Lord's victory. He is with you, O people of Judah and Jerusalem. [and you people reading *Full of Faith (or full of food?)*]. Do not be afraid or discouraged. Go out there tomorrow, for the Lord is with you! (2 Chronicles 20:l5-17, *New Living Translation*)

I became a blessing and I was blessed. Through increased clarity, my mode of behavior stabilized. My family life improved dramatically, my friendships flourished and I prospered in my employment, both financially and emotionally. It was God's amazing grace. He used my compassionate heart and willing spirit to talk and listen. Most often, I lived in contented abstinence, enjoying a calm dependence on God's ability, His goodness and his unfailing love, and I didn't overeat, no matter what was happening in my circumstances or how I felt.

...I am still not all I should be, but I am focusing all my energies on this one thing: Forgetting the past and looking forward to what lies ahead. I strain to reach the end of the race and receive the prize for which God, through Christ Jesus, is calling us up to heaven. (Philippians 3:13-14, *New Living Translation*)

Living Free

> ...I have learned to be content whatever the circumstances. I know what it is to be in need, and I know what it is to have plenty. I have learned the secret of being content in any and every situation, whether well fed or hungry, whether living in plenty or in want. I can do everything through him who gives me strength. (Philippians 4:11-13, *New International Version*)

The Christian looks *through* a problem, not *at* a problem. It was June 2001. I was happily rolling along, writing my book, telling people about Jesus and joyfully proclaiming freedom from food obsession and compulsive overeating. It had been over twelve years since my last binge. I had e-mail loops and many people looking to me for guidance. I was in my glory until my annual physical exam.

My doctor had ordered a bone density test as a standard procedure for a woman in her mid-forties. I razzed her, as if it was a waste of time, but she asked me to humor her and do it anyway. I was a model of good health, or so it seemed. After a minute's hesitation, hashing over the inconvenience of going to another appointment, I said, "Sure, I can do that," smugly believing the results would verify my admirable self-nurturing choices in life, plus it would supply impressive documentation for this book.

A week later, I got the shocking news, "You have osteoporosis. Your bones are frail. You only have 67% bone mass in your hip and 71% in your spine." It felt as if my heart fell to the floor with a splat. Angry with God, I yelled, "It's not fair! How can I tell people about you, Lord, if I am not well? What in the world do you expect of me?" I was also angry with the medical profession as I had done all the precautionary things to avoid osteoporosis, even hormone replacement therapy. *It's not fair. It's not fair. It's not fair.* I stomped my feet and had my tantrum.

God's timing is impeccable. A women's ministry breakfast was the following day. I spilled my guts to close friends at church, desperate for wisdom and comfort in my dismay. A cancer survivor sympathized with my pain and invited me to a seminar featuring a Christian natural health care professional, scheduled for the following weekend. Earlier I had scoffed at the need for such extreme measures. Health foods and supplements, organic vegetables and special foods were not for me. I thought they were all hogwash. My attitude held firm for years: "The medical profession and conventional nutritionists know best." This time, hope held my hand. I jumped on her bandwagon and without hesitation, I exclaimed, "Yes, I would love to go." We both laughed at my enthusiasm. It was a turnaround of extreme proportion.

After the seminar, I met with the specialist. I knew that God had set me up to hear a serious message: *dietary fats are necessary to distribute healthy nutrients throughout our bodies. Balance and moderation are necessary in all things.* Through the years, the media had encouraged reducing fats, which is wise. Extremists like me, however, went beyond what was reasonable. With the idea that less is best, many of us eliminated most dietary fat from our food plans. Experience is the best teacher. God got my attention with my new diagnosis of osteoporosis. I was ready to change.

The natural health care professional suggested the Zone Diet by Dr. Barry Sears. He developed a simple dietary plan to balance protein, carbohydrate and fat. I went home that night and combined my previous knowledge with the Zone philosophy. In other words, I modified the Zone Diet plan by eliminating all sugar, flour and wheat, and I set some bottom-lines as minimum daily requirements for my plan of eating. In time, I simplified my plan of eating and founded the Step Easy Food Plan.

My hope and my prayer is that I might help others avoid the potential hazard that could result because of unreasonable dietary restrictions of healthy fats in their food plans, and I trust that God will heal my body if it is His will.

> "For I know the plans I have for you," says the Lord. "They are plans for good and not for disaster, to give you a future and a hope." (Jeremiah 29:11, *New Living Translation*)

An Attitude of Gratitude

Live and love deeply, beyond food. God wants us to surrender our wills. He wants to use our hands, our mouths, our passions, our determined natures, our talents and our gifts to glorify Him and to edify the body of believers. He wants us to let go of our control, people pleasing, caretaking, anxiety, worry, negativity and fear. We walk in love. God directs our steps.

> Don't copy the behavior and customs of this world, but let God transform you into a new person by changing the way you think. Then you will know what God wants you to do, and you will know how good and pleasing and perfect his will really is. (Romans 12:2, *New Living Translation*)

I humbly share my experience, strength and hope in the Lord. Sharing the good news of His love and awesome ability keeps me excited. I have an attitude of gratitude. Whenever I get confounded, I ask Jesus what He would do, and I ask for His help in doing the right thing.

God is our refuge and strength, always ready to help in times of trouble. (Psalm 46:1, *New Living Translation*)

I wish I could tell you it is easy. I wish I could say I am successful 100% of the time. It is progress, not perfection. Hope for a better tomorrow sustains me. I am not where I want to be, but by the grace of God, I am not where I used to be. Striving toward the goal to be more like Jesus, I make an attempt each day to be all He wants and expects me to be. It is comforting to know that each new day offers another opportunity to "rise and shine." His mercies are new every single morning. (See Lamentations 3:23.)

When I am willing to listen to God, I am empowered. Letting go of my self-centered desires, I am content while waiting for God's plans to be revealed. I am confident that God will supply *all* my needs. (See Philippians 4:19) Scripture after Scripture imbedded in my heart soothes my brokenness, and I see glimpses of God's kingdom. I see righteousness, peace and joy in believing. (See Romans 14:17) Paul paints the picture of success. He shows us how to be happy. Do the right thing and be kind, loving, and respectful to others. Stop worrying and pray with an attitude of gratitude.

Always be full of joy in the Lord. I say it again—rejoice! Let everyone see that you are considerate in all you do. Remember, the Lord is coming soon. Don't worry about anything; instead, pray about everything. Tell God what you need, and thank him for all he has done. If you do this, you will experience God's peace, which is far more wonderful than the human mind can understand. His peace will guard your hearts and minds as you live in Christ Jesus. (Philippians 4:4-7, *New Living Translation*)

A Heart for God

Let us fix our eyes on Jesus, the author and perfecter of our faith, who for the joy set before him endured the cross, scorning its shame, and sat down at the right hand of the throne of God. (Hebrews 12:2, *New International Version*)

God taps me on the shoulder at 4:15 A.M. I hop out of bed. Groping for my eyeglasses, I am ready for a brand-new day. On my way to the bathroom, I begin my conversations with God. *Lord, You are faithful. Your love keeps me safe and strong. Thank You for loving me through yesterday. Please, Lord, help to see and do Your will today.*

I drop to my knees, "*Jesus, You are my all in all, the alpha and omega, the beginning and the end.*" I reflect upon the messages of His Word imbedded in the recesses of my mind. Seeking His will in my present circumstances, I am confident my answers will come. "*Thank You, Lord, for Your*

amazing grace. You have the capabilities of changing what
seems impossible. You are Lord, Savior, Prince of Peace,
Father God. I am blessed and empowered for another day.
Because of Your grace, I can be a blessing."

> Trust in the Lord and do good. Then you will live
> safely in the land and prosper. Take delight in the
> Lord, and he will give you your heart's desires.
> Commit everything you do to the Lord. Trust him,
> and he will help you. (Psalm 37:3-5, *New Living
> Translation*)

As I conclude the writing of *Sweet Surrender,* I reminisce to that summer evening so long ago when Jesus said, "Write a book. Tell the people about the gifts." It was the end of July in the year 2000. I had just celebrated twelve years of abstinence. *The Twelve Steps for Christians* Support Group had recently wrapped up another step study. Like the Israelites on the way to the Promised Land, I had traveled around and around the same mountain trudging in the wilderness. I sought truth amongst the lies. As God would have it, I grew steadily each time I was willing to surrender more character defects to the Lord. I surrendered control, caretaking, gossip, judgment, my messiah complex and the like. God carried me from glory to glory. My spirit gleamed with a passive, calm delight.

Carl and I were in a peaceful place. We were happy and secure. The boys were well and directed at school and at church. Life seemed better than ever. I felt as if the rough and rocky road of my past had been replaced. I was strolling through a beautiful garden, the kind that I have seen in home and garden magazines. Awestruck with my new life in Jesus, I bowed my head in humble adoration, "How can I best serve you, Lord Jesus?"

Joe and I sat perched in front of our television set one night; it served as the monitor for our internet service. I pulled rank as the mother, as I often did, and retrieved my e-mail messages first. Joe didn't mind. He sat in wait for his turn to go on-line half-watching, half-reading some book he had picked up at the Christian bookstore where he worked. One e-mail message hit me hard. I summoned Joe's attention, "Joe, did you read that sad story?" He shook his head as if to say, "No, it was none of my business." With mounting emotion, I told him that it was a food addict's desperate plea for help. I mumbled under my breath, "I remember those days, poor child. Lord, help her."

As I typed my response, Joe gained interest. Pouring out my heart and soul, I met the woman in her pain by rejoining some awful incidences in my past that looked ghastly at the time, but turned out to be pivotal pieces in God's perfect plan. In words I cannot remember now, I envisioned God carrying me on the wings of angels. My life is God's handiwork. I am perpetual work in progress.

> For we are God's masterpiece. He has created us anew in Christ Jesus, so that we can do the good things he planned for us long ago. (Ephesians 2:lo, *New Living Translation*)

Joe turned in my direction and said admirably, "Mom, you should write a book." I laughed aloud and dismissed the idea as absurd. Later, in my quiet time, I sat in contemplation. *Maybe Joe is right. Is this Your will for me, Lord? How in God's green earth am I going to do that?* My mind started clacking like a typewriter out of control spitting out page after page of gobbledygook.

By mere coincidence, of course, I am smiling because there are no accidents in God's world; Joe had just bought a used laptop computer from a friend at work. Joe, in his usual supportive way, offered to help me learn how to use it.

I chuckled for a couple of days imagining my future. It was almost inconceivable to grasp the whole concept. Joe was my sounding board. He kept my secret while I waited for the ideal time to "come out of the closet" with my "calling." It was only three days later when God told me that it was time to face the opposition. My battlefield started at home. Carl's disposition was objective and reasonable, but to me, he appeared negative, skeptical and more than doubtful. He was not an easy person to approach with "God talk."

Dare to Dream

> Now glory to God! By his mighty power at work within us, he is able to accomplish infinitely more than we would ever dare to ask or hope. (Ephesians 3:20, *New Living Translation*)

"Hampton Beach here we come." Carl, Joe and I headed for another summer vacation at the beach. Nervously I waited for the courage to announce my "assignment from God." In silence, I practiced my opening line, "Carl, God wants to use me..."

Carl will think it's bizarre. It is bizarre. I must be crazy. How am I going to write a book? Then, suddenly, out of the blue, my head stopped bashing God's instructions, and I heard in my spirit, "Just do it." My heart told me to be honest, open and willing to go to any lengths. *Who am I to say that God can't do this? Nothing is impossible with God. Okay, Lord, I am ready.*

With Joe in the backseat for moral support, I spouted in one quick breath, "Carl, God-asked-me-to-write-a-book." He looked at me half-smiling, half stunned. His expression said, "You have got to be kidding." Carl took a minute to process my proclamation. He presented my obvious handicap: "Pam, because you don't read, except books about God and nutrition, you certainly don't have a diversified vocabulary. How do you expect to write a book?" More boldly than I imagined, I said, "God wouldn't ask me to do something without giving me the skills to do it." This time he laughed aloud.

Although Carl had learned not to argue with my determined will, his body language expressed serious apprehension. Unable to contain his smirk, he challenged, "Okay, what are you going to write about?" I briefly explained that I was planning to write about my life and the gifts I had received along the way. Silence followed for what seemed like an eternity.

Swallowing my insecurities, I tried to break the ice. Lightheartedly I said, "Come on; help me think of a name for the book." As we joked back and forth about possibilities, Carl's tender heart started to surface. He was rough around the edges, but soft and sweet on the inside. He reflected upon some of our milestones and then concluded, "We certainly have had our ups and downs through the years; they were like bumps in the road of life." We agreed that God's love carried us over some exceptionally rough and rocky roads. The title, *Just Another Bump in the Road,* won our votes.

We arrived at our cottage. I hurriedly unpacked my gear. Blindly I sat at the outdated laptop. Except for e-mail, I was computer illiterate, but God used Joe's calm spirit to quietly instruct me in computer lingo. Joe had the patience of a saint. God bless him. Hours later, I finally understood enough to write and save my messages.

I typed up a storm rambling through my early life, until God said, "Stop. I want you to tell people about your changing faith. Tell them about your food addiction, your 'turnaround.'" As I waited to announce my latest "word from God," I came up with a new title, *Faith-ful (or full of food?).* By the grace of God, my life was full of faith, and no longer full of food.

Carl continued to watch and listened with an amused glimmer in his eyes. He may have thought I was in fantasyland, but he saw me happily toddling along. That was all that mattered to him. If I was happy, he was happy.

There were many "bumps in the road" along the way to finishing *Full of Faith (or full of food?)*. I am here to tell you that every breath in this book is a gift from the Lord. Miracles happen. I know because I am one and this book is another. There is no way in the world I could have done this work without God's help. I am confident that God who began a good work in me will be faithful to complete it. (See Philippians 1:6)

My heart and soul cries out to you, beloved friend, "Taste and see that the Lord is good; blessed is the man who takes refuge in him." (Psalm 34:8, *New International Version*) *Use my words, Lord Jesus, if it is Your will, to touch someone, somewhere, if only with a thimbleful of hope or an ounce of love.* I wish I could spoon-feed every lost, lame, limping one and distraught food addict alike. It is time for me to "let go and let God." Into His hands, I place my trust, my confident expectation and my hope. God bless you and keep you safe until we meet again on earth or in heaven.

> I pray that Christ will be more and more at home in your hearts as you trust in him. May your roots go down deep into the soil of God's marvelous love. And may you have the power to understand, as all God's people should, how wide, how long, how high, and how deep his love really is. May

you experience the love of Christ, though it is so great you will never fully understand it. Then you will be filled with the fullness of life and power that comes from God.

Now glory to God! By his mighty power at work within us, he is able to accomplish infinitely more than we would ever dare to ask or hope. May he be given glory in the church and in Christ Jesus forever and ever through endless ages. Amen. (Ephesians 3:17-21, *New Living Translation*)

The Long and Winding Road

"There is an appointed time for everything. And there is a time for every event under heaven..." Ecclesiastes 3:1 NAS

Never Give up

"Let us not become weary in doing good, for at the proper time we will reap a harvest if we do not give up." Galatians 6:9 NIV

As I sat watching the movie, "Conversations with God" with a recovering food addict/friend., I cried through the man's journey, but then heard God say to me, almost audibly, "It's time."

It's finally time. I waited almost ten years to hear those words. "It's time for what, Lord?"

Time to share the good news of recovery through meetings, an interactive blog, flyers to churches, posters in church halls or on grocery store bulletin boards. It's time.

Years ago, I heard over and over again "build it and they will come." I thought God meant NOW (at that time), but I am seeing today that I had more to learn. I needed more experience, more strength, more hope, more faith. I was at the growing-mustard-seed phase of life.

> "For every house is built by someone, but God is the builder of everything." (Hebrews 3:5 NIV)

I am not saying that I have arrived, not at all, but I am ready and willing to step out and see if God parts the sea, so to speak. He didn't part the Red Sea until Moses stepped into it. I won't know if this ministry will grow unless I step out in faith and do my 1%.

"God, bless it or block it. Your will, not mine, be done."

A Sweet Surrender

> "Do not conform to the patterns of this world, but be transformed by the renewing of your mind. Then you will be able to test and approve what God's will is--His good, pleasing and perfect will." Romans 12:2 NIV

On July 23rd, 2013, I celebrated 25 years of freedom from compulsive and addictive eating. Grace of an amazing God.

Until recently, *Full of Faith* was left dormant, almost kicked to the curb. I kept the website through the years, but didn't expect much. The hope of doing more with it had vanished. I accepted that I had misunderstood God's plan and purpose for my life, and I was okay being wife, mother, grandmother, daycare provider and an active member of my 12-step support groups.

Then a motivator and encourager started writing to me. Karen S from Florida told me that my website and the book, Full of Faith (or full of food?) had touched her heart back in 2006. Her gentle persuasion inspired me to do more.

Besides my traditional 12-step fellowship, I was one of the founding fathers of Christian Food Addicts in Recovery (christianfoodaddicts.weebly.com). There are other Christian fellowships, too, that have popped up through the years. Pat N has ongoing meetings (bibleforfood.org), Stephanie from MA (bible4recovery.com) and Mary from MA (faithfulsurrender.com) also have meetings for Christian 12-steppers. These support groups satisfied my need to be with other Christian addicts in recovery.

Full of Faith (or full of food?)

Seeking nutritional knowledge is still my second-nature. I read the latest research on what's healthy and what's not, and I have incorporated some of my new-found insights into my food plan (with the help of God and my sponsor).

Sometime around my 20th year anniversary of abstinence, the hidden promises came true for me. My way of eating became as easy as breathing. It's who I am. It became my way of life.

"We feel as though we had been placed in a position of neutrality--safe and protected. We have not even sworn off. Instead, the problem has been removed. It does not exist for us. We are neither cocky nor are we afraid. This is our experience. That is how we react as long as we keep in fit spiritual condition." (Alcoholics Anonymous, page 85)

Today my food plan is unique and right for my nutritional needs. I still treat my food like a prescription drug, but have a sponsor/accountability partner who trusts that I have intelligent reasoning. This is my food plan at this time, but it might not be this way forever:

breakfast

6 oz. plain non-fat yogurt

1 oz. oatmeal or oatbran (measured dry, then cooked with 1/2 cup water)

1 egg or 3 oz. cottage cheese

2 tablespoon ground flax seeds

7 raw almonds (I do not eat roasted or salted nuts or seeds)

lunch

3 oz. protein or 6 oz beans

16 oz. vegetables (usually 8 oz. cooked, 8 oz. salad)

2 tablespoons salad dressing (no sugar)

1 heaping tablespoon raw sunflower seeds

1 heaping teaspoon nutritional yeast

1 heaping teaspoon chia seeds

5 oz. berries or 1 medium sized fruit

dinner

3 oz. protein or 6 oz. beans

16 oz. vegetables (usually 8 oz. cooked, 8 oz. salad)

2 tablespoons salad dressing (no sugar)

4 oz. potato or 6 oz. butternut squash

1 tablespoon butter

l heaping tablespoon raw sunflower seeds

1 heaping teaspoon nutritional yeast

1 heaping teaspoon chia seeds

6 oz. plain non-fat yogurt

1 tablespoon ground flax seeds

7 raw almonds

When I go to a restaurant, I typically order a salad entree with grilled chicken, shrimp or steak on top. I order a side of cooked vegetables and if it's dinner time, I order a baked potato (sweet if it's available). I cut the potato in half, and add a pat of butter. I bring my salad dressing or I measure olive oil in a teaspoon (3 teaspoons equals a Tablespoon).

I am not suggesting this food plan for anyone. I am sharing how my food plan has evolved through the years. This plan works for me. I maintain my goal weight, my blood work is phenomenal, and I am satisfied.

This Little Light of Mine

"Fit spiritual condition" is the key that keeps my program "green"--alive and growing.

God is the answer, what's the question? Instead of telling God how big my problems are, I tell my problems how big my God is. Prayer changes things.

These are not new thoughts, just more firmly secured in my heart, mind and emotions today. My daily routine has changed through the years, too. Each morning, I always start the day in prayer. I seek God's face. I love and adore Him. I thank God for my blessings, then I pray for myself, my husband (Carl) and each of our children (Dan and Heather, Joe and Stacy) and our grandchildren (Caleb, Isaac and Anna) individually, with specifics.

I pray for my daycare children, others in need, and for the Christian 12-step fellowships.

Later, after I do my morning walk, I jump on a phone meeting while eating my weighed and measured breakfast.

I read a small portion of the Bible and text my thoughts to some people who are reading along with me. It's an encouraging interchange.

After lunch, I have a dedicated quiet time, a time to sit with God, be present, experience Him.

Before bed, I do a tenth step inventory. With the hope of being God-pleasing, I examine my thoughts and attitude during my day's interactions. If I need to apologize for an inappropriate word or deed, I take note and follow-through as it is God's will.

I'm Gonna Let It Shine

Preach always and if necessary use words.

I am happy that I learned to feel my feelings. I now experience a full array of emotions. I cry, I laugh. My smile is real. When I came into program, I not only used food to fix a feeling, but I used people to fill the emptiness in my heart-- my co-dependency was a huge issue. Yikes and ouch!

Letting my children grow up, leave home, get married was a struggle beyond my comprehension, but God took my hand and led me through my bewilderment. I didn't die and my boys are wonderful children of God. They both married lovely women, and I have three amazing grandchildren. This is the life God rewards.

My husband and I are forever working on our marriage. I am learning to apply the lessons of many Christian self-help books that have taken part in my better-than-before relationship with my husband. It's not so much about him, but about me and my attitude. When I place him (and everyone else) in the hands of God, I enjoy my life. I have made a lot of steps in the right direction, but I am holding on to hope of better days still to come.

Let it Shine

> "You did not choose me. I chose you and appointed you so that you might bear fruit that will last..." (John 15:16 NIV)

On September 22, 2013, Karen S from Florida officially joined the Full of Faith ministry.

"Two are better than one..."

If it's God's will, we hope to link with foodaddictioninstitute.org in sharing the hope of recovery with people who struggle with overeating, under eating, eating addictively, have warped body images or whatever separates them from experiencing the full measure of God's love.

May we continue to grow in love, truth and understanding.

"Whom the son has set free is free indeed!" (John 8:36)

Chapter Five

Recovery—A Way of Life

"Whether you turn to the right or to the left, your
ears will hear a voice behind you, saying, 'This is
the way; walk in it.'"

(Isaiah 30:21, New International Version)

Pot of Gold

One night, I had a dream. I saw a perplexed person,
with no face or size, staring into a dark tunnel. The person
was holding a flashlight in one hand and a map in the other.
God told me that the map is the Twelve Steps, the flashlight
represents willingness, and the tunnel is God's will and His
love. In order to find recovery, we walk through the tunnel,
where we find God's guidance and compassion.

I picture many people looking into the tunnel, but
stopping in their tracks. Some say, "It's too hard" or "I'm not
that bad." They may say, "Life is okay. The grass is green

enough," thus accepting what I call "tolerable recovery". We have options. God gives us free will, but He also offers us gifts. On the other side of the tunnel, there are beautiful gardens beyond our imaginations!

Every time I put down a problem food or let go of another character flaw, I walk through yet another tunnel. Recovery is ongoing. Whatever the struggle, God never brings you to it without bringing you through it. I will keep my flashlight in hand and carry my map, along with my Bible, and walk until God brings me to my next tunnel. Thy will, not mine, be done.

It's Electric

> What is faith? It is the confident assurance that something we want is going to happen. It is the certainty that what we hope for is waiting for us, even though we cannot see it up ahead. (Hebrews 11:1, *The Living Bible*)

Sometimes I stumble in the dark groping for the light switch. When I find it, I fully expect the lights to go on as I flip the switch. Although I cannot see the wires in the wall or the current traveling through them, nor do I understand the technical application, I believe in electricity. It is a proven fact to me. If I switch the light off, I sit in the dark. Switch it on, I see. Faith is believing in your heart and knowing the truth. Jesus reveals Himself to His children through the Holy Spirit.

> ...Jesus said to the people, "I am the Light of the world. So if you follow me, you won't be stumbling through the darkness, for living light will flood your path." (John 8:12, *The Living Bible*)

Can you imagine the day when Noah started building the ark? God asked him to design and build a huge boat on dry land. Strange as it may have sounded, Noah heard the command and began the work. People thought he was crazy, but faith carried him. The mission was peculiar, but he continued. We all know how this story unfolds. God held the master plan. Noah and his family lived while the others perished in the flood.

The world is full of people voicing their opinions. The media tells us what to do, what to wear and what to think. It is time to stand up and focus on God, who is the true source of love, wisdom and power. We find peace, serenity and joy when we let go of our fears and trust God.

> Peace I leave with you; My [own] peace I now give *and* bequeath to you. Not as the world gives do I give to you. Do not let your hearts be troubled, neither let them be afraid. [Stop allowing yourselves to be agitated and disturbed; and do

not permit yourselves to be fearful and intimidated and cowardly and unsettled.] (John 14:27, *Amplified Bible*)

The Serenity Prayer with Scripture

The Serenity Prayer guides us into right thinking when we struggle with the ebb and flow of life. Scripture affirmations reinforce the truth that sets us free one day at a time.

> All Scripture is inspired by God and is useful to teach us what is true and to make us realize what is wrong in our lives. It straightens us out and teaches us to do what is right. It is God's way of preparing us in every way, fully equipped for every good thing God wants us to do. (2 Timothy 4:16-17, *New Living Translation*)

God, grant me the serenity

> Don't worry about anything; instead, pray about everything. Tell God what you need, and thank him for all he has done. If you do this, you will experience God's peace, which is far more wonderful than the human mind can understand. His peace will guard your hearts and minds as you live in Christ Jesus. (Philippians 4:6-7, *New Living Translation*)

To accept the things I cannot change,

> ...I have learned how to be content (satisfied to the point where I am not disturbed or disquieted)

in whatever state I am. (Philippians 4:11, *Amplified Bible*)

The courage to change the things I can,

Commit everything you do to the Lord. Trust him to help you do it, and he will. (Psalm 37:5, *The Living Bible*)

And the wisdom to know the difference,

Lean on, trust in *and* be confident in the Lord with all your heart *and* mind and do not rely on your own insight *or* understanding. In all your ways know, recognize, *and* acknowledge Him, and He will direct *and* make straight *and* plain your paths. (Proverbs 3:5-6, *Amplified Bible*)

Living one day at a time,

The steadfast love of the Lord never ceases, his mercies never come to an end. They are new every morning; great is thy faithfulness. (Lamentations 3:22-23, *Revised Standard Version*)

Enjoying one moment at a time,

This is the day that the Lord has made; let us rejoice and be glad in it. (Psalm 118:24, *New International Version)*

Accepting hardship as a pathway to peace;

God is our refuge and strength, an ever-present help in trouble. (Psalm 46:1, *New International Version)*

Taking, as Jesus did, this sinful world as it is, not as I would have it;

> We are pressed on every side by troubles, but we are not crushed and broken. We are perplexed, but we don't give up and quit. We are hunted down, but God never abandons us. We get knocked down, but we get up again and keep going. (2 Corinthians 4:8-9, *New Living Translation*)

Trusting that You will make all things right if I surrender to your will;

> We know that God causes everything to work together for the good of those who love God and are called according to his purpose for them. (Romans 8-28, *New Living Translation*)

So that I may be reasonably happy in this life

> The Lord is my strength, my shield from every danger. I trust in him with all my heart. He helps me, and my heart is filled with joy... (Psalm 28:7, *New Living Translation*)

And supremely happy with You forever in the next. Amen.

> Surely goodness and love will follow me all the days of my life, and I will dwell in the house of the Lord forever. (Psalm 23:6, *New International Version*)

> For God so greatly loved *and* dearly prized the world that He [even] gave up His only begotten (unique) Son, so that whoever believes in (trusts

in, clings to, relies on) Him shall not perish (come to destruction, be lost) but have eternal (everlasting) life. (John 3:16, *Amplified Bible)*

Heart to Heart—Are You a Food Addict Like Me?

And you will know the truth, and the truth will set you free. (John 8:32, *New Living Translation*)

If you want to live free from compulsive overeating and food obsession, strap on your seatbelt and get ready for the ride of your life! Realization, acceptance and surrender are the first steps. Take some time when you are not rushed and write your thoughts in response to each of the following questions.

What is your goal? Unconsciously I had a fantasy that thin people were emotionally stable and happy people, who were lovable and loved. Today I know that thin is just thin. It is not always the result of emotional or physical health. Examine your expectations. If you succeeded on a diet and reached your goal weight, how would this accomplishment change your life?

Do you feed a feeling? Do you automatically turn to food to fix a broken heart or a wounded spirit? As a child, did you learn to respond to feelings of happiness and sadness with excess food? List the family members who influenced your relationship with food.

Note that many food addicts come from dysfunctional families. In recovery, we learn that it is okay to love our families while accepting the fact that some of our closest relationships were not always physically, emotionally or spiritually healthy.

Who is your God? People say that whatever occupies most of a person's thought-life is their God. Do you wake up in the morning thinking about food, think about it during your daily activities and go to bed thinking about food?

Many people who struggle with overeating, poor body image and food obsession try many different avenues in search of a solution. What weight loss techniques have you tried through the years? Make a list of doctors, diet and exercise programs, pills, hypnotists and the like and talk about the benefits and deficits of each program.

Do you think that self-control through behavior modification is the answer to recovery from *compulsive** overeating and food addiction?

*Compulsive is a term that describes an act outside of our will. We want to do what is right but cannot resist the very thing that we know causes us harm. It is a downward slide. In the advanced stages of food addiction, an overeater takes one compulsive bite and then loses control, more or less, depending on the individual's progression of the disease.

...No matter which way I turn, I can't make myself do right. I want to, but I can't. (Romans 7:18, *New Living Translation*)

Do you agree that compulsive overeating and food addiction is a physical, emotional and spiritual malady just like alcoholism?

Are you ready to say "yes" to life and "no" to excess food today?"

My rendition of steps one, two and three is, "I am powerless over food. Despite intelligent reasoning and a determined will to stop overeating, I cannot do it without dependence on God. Lord, I surrender. Give me wisdom and willingness to succeed today where I have failed previously."

Smile. This is a one-day-at-a-time, one-step-at-a-time program. The disease of food addiction is debilitating, progressive and ultimately fatal, however, through the amazing love and grace of God, we offer you a solution. Through shared experiences of like-minded people, the disease can be arrested one day at a time.

You've Got a Friend

"Help! Somebody, please help me! I have fallen and I can't get up." The poor chap had fallen into a pit. A doctor answers the cries with intelligent reasoning. He writes a prescription and throws it into the hole, but to no avail. The painful moans continue, "Please, God, help me! Isn't there somebody who can help me?" A pastor wanders by, scribbles a prayer on a piece of paper, and throws it into the hole. Still more groans, "Woe is me! Help me. Somebody help me!" A kind stranger walks by and immediately jumps into the hole. The troubled soul yells in disbelieve, "Are you crazy? Now we are both stuck in this hole!" With an assuring smile, the gentleman replies, "Trust me, my friend. I've been here before. I know the way out."

Twelve-step programs create a circle of love. We find love and then pass the torch. We love others. It is a blessing and a joy to share our experience, strength and hope with those still suffering.

> Two are better than one... If one falls down, his friend can help him up. But pity the man who falls and has no one to help him up! Though one may be overpowered, two can defend themselves. A cord of three strands is not quickly broken. (Ecclesiastes 4:9-10, 12, *New International Version*)

The Little Engine that Could

"Mommy, I can't do it!" Daniel stomped out of the room frustrated once again. He had repeatedly tried to tie his shoes. I wanted to teach him, to instruct and guide him. He was stubborn. He was just like me. Demanding independence, he'd yell, "I CAN DO IT MYSELF!" I sat and watched him tangle the laces, twisting them, twirling them in and out, up and down. I waited for him to ask for help. It was a long, hard road. In time, he surrendered and let me teach him the skills he lacked. Desire and determination were not enough.

The same theory applies to recovery from food addiction. People want to diet. They set their minds toward the goal of being thin and sane, but they cannot stop overeating. When a person understands addiction and says, "Yes, I am a food addict. I surrender." He or she needs to learn how to arrest the disease. Compassionate people, who have experienced success, are anxious to help. It is obvious, however, that we are unique, and people come with different needs. With patient perseverance and open communication, each person can grow beyond the disease into a happy, joyful life.

Teachers, guides, mentors, helping hands, sponsors, whatever the title, they are a necessary piece of the puzzle to get well. People need people to shine a light in the darkness. God has magnificently designed a plan for each of His children. The suffering, afflicted ones can come together and find God's care and protection. We can comfort the brokenhearted, announce liberty to captives (those actively overeating), and open the eyes of the blind (Christians who are uninformed about eating disorders and food addicts lacking faith).

> ...the time of God's favor to them has come...he will give: beauty for ashes; joy instead of mourning; praise instead of heaviness. (Isaiah 61:2-3, *The Living Bible*)

Slow and Steady Wins the Race

One courageous day, I stepped out of my isolation and faced my addiction. It was the first step to a changed life. I learned about addictive behavior by listening to people in recovery. I cried with them, rejoiced with them and witnessed new life in them. Hope arose in my spirit. I was not alone anymore.

If you want what we have, we offer helpful tools as options to consider. They are not rules, requirements or regulations, simply what has worked for other food addicts and compulsive overeaters. Always pray for guidance. Be honest, open and willing to listen. God sets the pace. Slow and steady wins the race.

Food Plan:

> Blessed are those who hunger and thirst for righteousness, for they will be filled. (Matthew 5:6, *New International Version*)

To live free from overeating, it is important to make a decision (a firm commitment) to follow a specific, disciplined plan of eating. Although there can be "different strokes for different folks," most long-term recovering food addicts avoid sugar, flour and foods that trigger a craving.

We feel that *God and abstinence are the most important things, without exception.* The Bible teaches us that nothing can separate us from the love of God (1); our ties to Him are not contingent on what we do (2), but on simple, childlike faith (3). However, we feel separated from God the minute we say, "Yes" to some "forbidden fruit." When Eve listened to the serpent in the Garden of Eden, her relationship with God changed the moment she ate that enticing apple. It was not her food. In abstinence, we can see more clearly what God wants us to do, and we can enjoy the fruits of believing (5).

> The Kingdom of God is not a matter of what we eat or drink, but of living a life of goodness and peace and joy in the Holy Spirit (Romans 14:17, *New Living Translation)*

See (l) Romans 7-8, (2) Ephesians 2:8-9, (3) Luke 18:17, (4) Genesis 3:1-8, (5) Galatians 5:22-23.

Prayer and Meditation:

> [Jesus said,] Ask and it will be given to you; seek and you will find; knock and the door will be opened to you. (Matthew 7:7, *New International Version*)

To stay connected to the only true source of strength, we dedicate a specific time in the morning, before we begin the hustle and bustle of the day, to pray and meditate. This gives us the opportunity to bring all our thoughts and concerns to the Lord. We seek His guidance and direction. Jesus sent the Holy Spirit as the: "Comforter, Counselor, Helper, Intercessor, Advocate, Strengthener, and Standby." (John 14:16, *Amplified Bible*) And He taught us how to pray:

> When you pray, go away by yourself, shut the door behind you, and pray to your Father secretly. Then your Father, who knows all secrets, will reward you...your Father knows exactly what you need even before you ask him! (Matthew 6:6-8, *New Living Translation*)

Prayer Partners/Friends in Recovery (i.e., Sponsors):

Most food addicts contact one or more persons daily on the telephone or through the Internet. We find freedom when we commit our intended plan of eating to another person(s) in recovery each new day. Beyond food, people in recovery share a mutual desire to seek and do God's will. Bonds are tightly woven as we pray together for knowledge and wisdom in all our affairs.

> Two are better than one, because they have a good return for their work: If one falls down, his friend can help him up. But pity the man who falls and has no one to help him up! Though one may be overpowered, two can defend themselves. A cord of three strands is not quickly broken. (Ecclesiastes 4:9-10, 12, *New International Version*)

Face-to-Face and Phone Meetings:

> Where two or three come together in my name, there am I with them. (Matthew 18:20, *New International Version*)

Meetings are gatherings of two or more like-minded people who come together to share their experience, strength and hope in recovery. Fellowship with other addicts gives us the opportunity to identify our common concerns, and we share the gifts we receive through the program.

Twelve-Step Christian Support Group:

Christian Food Addicts in Recovery phone meetings
www.Christianfoodaddicts.weebly.com.
Bibleforfood.org

Bible4recovery.com

faithfulsurrender.com

fulloffaith.com

Traditional Twelve-Step Support Groups for Compulsive Overeaters and Food Addicts:

CEA/HOW (Compulsive Overeaters Anonymous/HOW)

FAA (Food Addicts Anonymous)

OA (Overeaters Anonymous)

RFA (Recovery from Food Addiction)

Check the telephone directory, the newspaper or the Internet for face-to-face meetings near you. Phone meetings are listed on group web sites.

The Telephone:

The telephone is an easily accessible mode of communication that helps us to handle the highs and lows we all experience. We can "reach out and touch someone" instead of reaching for the food, which is no longer a viable option.

The Internet:

The Internet provides light to a diverse audience. From coast to coast, people with addictions share their experience, strength and hope in recovery. People attend various 12-step meetings on-line, go to chat rooms, and obtain vast information about the different aspects of recovery. Visit my web site: www.fulloffaith.com for an up-to-date view of my personal interests

Literature:

> Open my eyes to see wonderful things in your Word. I am but a pilgrim here on earth: how I need a map—and your commands are my chart and guide. I long for your instructions more than I can tell. (Psalm 119:18-20, *The Living Bible*)

The Bible is our ultimate source and guide. However, *Alcoholics Anonymous* supplies easily identifiable keys to recovery from addictive behavior, and daily devotionals are helpful to maintain progress in the program. Many recovering addicts read three books each day: *The Holy Bible*, a page of *Alcoholics Anonymous* and a daily devotional, maybe *Twenty-Four Hours a Day*, plus other 12-step recovery literature as their quest for knowledge and truth increases.

Recommended reading:

Alcoholics Anonymous, third edition, New York: Alcoholics Anonymous, World Service, 1976

Bariatric Surgery and Food Addiction, Preoperative Considerations Copyright 2009, by Philip R. Werdell M. A.

Food Addiction Recovery, A New Model of Professional Support - The ACORN Primary Intensive with Mary Foushi and Clare Weldon, Copyright 2007 by Philip R. Werdell,

Food Addiction: The Body Knows by Kay Sheppard, Health Communications, Inc. (Revised l993, 1989)

The Life Recovery Bible, Tyndale House Publishers, Inc. (1998)

The Twelve Steps for Christians, Revised Edition by Friends in Recovery, RPI Publishing, Inc. (1994)

Twenty-Four Hours a Day, Hazelden Foundation (1975)

Why Can't I Stop Eating? Recognizing, Understanding and Overcoming Food Addiction, by Danowski and Lazaro

For professional help, go to: http://foodaddiction.com/wp-content/uploads/acorn_brochure.pdf

Writing:

Most food addicts write a committed food plan each new day. Some people write in a food journal and some write to one of our internet e-mail loops. Either way, when we make a commitment, it releases the obsession to entertain food thoughts. We plan what we do and do what we plan. People in recovery often say, "People who fail to plan, plan to fail."

We also write fourth-step inventories and periodic entries in a journal. When we put our thoughts and feelings on paper, it opens the lines of communication to God. Writing a list of our daily blessings helps us to acknowledge the gifts we receive. On a bleak day, we reflect back and live each day with an attitude of gratitude.

Love and Service:

> ....Love your neighbor as yourself. (Galatians 5:14, *New International Version*)

Bill Wilson, founder of Alcoholics Anonymous, told us that "love and service" kept him sober. The same theory works for all addictions. When we extend our hearts and hands to other people, we become a reflection of God's love.

We can show up at meetings, make a phone call or help a newcomer get started in the program, or we can call a friend or family member to say, "I care about you." Maybe volunteer to help at a nursing home, a homeless shelter or a hospital. There are always people in need of a gentle smile or a word of encouragement. The key is to reach out and share the good news of Jesus in simple acts of kindness. By our examples, we are "salt and light" to the world. (See Matthew 5:13-16)

Confidentiality and Respect:

> Do for others what you would like them to do for you... (Matthew 7:12, *New Living Translation*)

Refraining from criticism and gossip, we accept that we are people striving toward recovery. We are all equal in God's eyes.

> Don't just pretend that you love others; really love them. Hate what is wrong. Stand on the side of good. Love each other with brotherly affection and take delight in honoring each other... Work happily together. Don't try to act big. Don't try to get into the good graces of important people, but enjoy the company of ordinary folks. And don't think you know it all! (Romans 12:9-10,16, *The Living Bible*)

Spiritual Training and Encouragement

Church: To grow in spiritual matters, it is helpful to attend a Christ-centered church. A healthy church provides a well-rounded diet of Christian education through the messages presented at weekly services, Bible studies and small group ministries. Fellowship is instrumental in understanding living faith.

Television and Radio Ministries: We can benefit through practical teaching of God's Word in the comfort of our own homes. Personally, I have found some rich and rewarding messages in the ministries of *Life in the Word* with Joyce Meyer, *In Touch* with Charles Stanley, *Focus on the Family* with James Dobson and *Family and Marriage Today* with Jimmy and Karen Evans.

Christian Music:

We listen to music that soothes our spirits in times of trouble and directs our minds to righteousness, peace and joy in believing.

Physical Exercise:

It is wise to incorporate some form of physical fitness as a part of a daily routine. Walking is a common choice. It is easy to do, requires no special equipment beyond sneakers, and it easily fits into most lifestyles. Bike riding, canoeing, volleyball and strolls on the beach are fun activities. When we need to rake leaves or shovel snow, we try to consider the health benefits, instead of the chore. Asking God for help, we make an effort to incorporate exercise into our everyday lives.

The Elevator is Broken—Try the Steps

God introduced me to a 12-step recovery program for my food addiction; He blessed me with freedom from compulsive overeating and food obsession. In my clarity of mind, without excess food, I began to see other areas of my life that needed healing. I welcomed the opportunity to understand God's instructions from reading his Word. *The Twelve Steps for Christians* supplied the map of the Bible for sustaining the highest quality of life, which is peaceful, happy, joyful existence on earth.

> And so, dear brothers and sisters, I plead with you to give your bodies to God. Let them be a living and holy sacrifice—the kind he will accept. When you think of what he has done for you, is this too much to ask? Don't copy the behavior and customs of this world, but let God transform you into a new person by changing the way you think. Then you will know what God wants you to do, and you will know how good and pleasing and perfect his will really is. (Romans 12:1-2, *New Living Translation*)

Acknowledgment of my powerlessness, and the very real fact that I only knew what I knew, were the baby steps to healing. As I remained abstinent from sugar and flour each new day, I began to see God's will in my life.

I learned *how to love and accept love.*

I learned *that calm, respectful tones of communication worked.*

I learned the skills necessary to respond in appropriate ways when annoyances and resentments flooded my thinking.

I learned to face my fears and work through them.

I learned to replace negativity with positive, life-giving affirmations.

I learned to stop manipulating and controlling people.

I learned that people are worthy of their opinions. It was okay if someone had a different opinion than mine. It didn't make them "good" or "right" and me "bad" or "wrong."

I learned to properly and respectfully take care of myself.

 I learned that inappropriate behavior was not acceptable from anyone.

I learned to accept and use criticism in a positive, constructive way.

I learned that I was worthy of love and respect.

What people thought of me was none of my business. I had to be willing to listen and admit,

time and time again, that I didn't know what I didn't know.

In God's time, with His constant help, I grew to understand and love myself and enjoy God's perfect plan for my life. I began to accept life on life's terms. I learned to trust God in everything, knowing that He was guiding my recovery.

The 12-step program works if you "work" it, although it is not always easy. Physical, emotional and spiritual healing requires patience, perseverance, love, understanding, commitment and accountability. You will find joy unspeakable if you apply these principles to your life. I didn't say, "You *might* find joy unspeakable." I said, "You *will* find joy unspeakable" through God's amazing grace!

If you open your hearts and minds to God's perfect plan, and focus your attention on Him, your life will continue to have more and more quality. Peace, joy and unfailing love will follow you everywhere.

> Blessed (happy, enviably fortunate, and spiritually prosperous—possessing the happiness produced by the experience of God's favor and especially conditioned by the revelation of His grace, regardless of their outward conditions) are the

pure in heart, for they shall see God! [Ps.24:3,4] (Matthew 5:8, *Amplified Bible*)

The Twelve Steps and Relevant Scripture

Step 1: We admitted we were powerless over our food addiction—that our lives had become unmanageable.

> I am completely discouraged—I lie in the dust... (Psalm 119:25, *The Living Bible)*

Step 2: Came to believe that a Power greater than ourselves could restore us to sanity.

> Open my eyes to see wonderful things in your Word. I am but a pilgrim here on earth: how I need a map—and your commands are my chart and guide. I long for your instructions more than I can tell. (Psalm 119:18-20, *The Living Bible*)

Step 3: Made a decision to turn our will and our lives over to the care of God, *as we understood Him.*

> Trust in the Lord with all your heart and lean not on your own understanding; in all your ways acknowledge him, and he will make your paths straight. (Proverbs 3:5-6, New International Version)

Step 4: Made a searching and fearless moral inventory of ourselves.

> Let every person carefully scrutinize *and* examine *and* test his own conduct *and* his own work...(Galatians 6:4, *Amplified Bible*)

Step 5: Admitted to God, to ourselves, and to another human being the exact nature of our wrongs.

Confess to one another therefore your faults (your slips, your false steps, your offenses, your sins) and pray [also] for one another, that you may be healed... (James 5:16, *Amplified Bible*)

Step 6: Were entirely ready to have God remove all these defects of character.

Do not resent it when God chastens and corrects you, for his punishment is proof of his love. Just as a father punishes a son he delights in to make him better, so the Lord corrects you. (Proverbs 3:11-12, *The Living Bible*)

Step 7: Humbly asked Him to remove our shortcomings.

But if we confess our sins to him, he can be depended on to forgive us and to cleanse us from every wrong... (1 John 1:9, *The Living Bible*)

Step 8: Made a list of all persons we had harmed, and became willing to make amends to them all.

Do to others as you would have them do to you. (Luke 6:31, *New International Version)*

Step 9: Made direct amends to such people wherever possible, except when to do so would injure them or others.

Bear with each other and forgive whatever grievances you may have against one another. Forgive as the Lord forgave you. (Colossians 3:13, *New International Version*)

Step 10: Continued to take personal inventory and when we were wrong promptly admitted it.

Now your attitudes and thoughts must all be constantly changing for the better. Yes, you must be a new and different person, holy and good. Clothe yourself with this new nature. Stop lying to each other; tell the truth, for we are parts of each other and when we lie to each other we are hurting ourselves. (Ephesians 4:23-25, *The Living Bible*)

Step 11: Sought through prayer and meditation to improve our conscious contact with God, *as we understood Him*, praying only for knowledge of His will for us and the power to carry that out.

Pray all the time. Ask God for anything in line with the Holy Spirit's wishes. Plead with him, reminding him of your needs, and keep praying earnestly for all Christians everywhere. (Ephesians 6:18, *New Living Translation*)

Step 12: Having had a spiritual awakening as the result of these steps, we tried to carry this message to food addicts, and to practice these principles in all our affairs.

It is God himself, in his mercy, who has given us this wonderful work [of telling his Good News to others] and so we never give up. (2 Corinthians 4:1, *The Living Bible*)

Permission to use the Twelve Steps of Alcoholics Anonymous® for adaptation granted by AA World Services, Inc

Chapter Six

Food Plans/Abstinence

Plan What You Do and Do What You Plan

"Everything is permissible—but not everything is beneficial..."

(1 Corinthians 10:23, *New International Version*)

Different Strokes for Different Folks

Freedom from overeating and food obsession is the goal. A *healthy* body is an obvious manifestation of success. However, many find other surprising benefits when they surrender to the disease of food addiction. They recognize a peace that passes all understanding, and in time, they find happiness and joy in trusting God each new day.

"When the Holy Spirit controls our lives he will produce this kind of fruit in us: love, joy, peace, patience, kindness, goodness, faithfulness, gentleness and self-control..." (Galatians 5:22-23, *The Living Bible*)

The recovery solution for overeating is a controversial subject. There are many opinions and many sources of information. My personal experience taught me to investigate the possibilities. I asked God to help me discern the truth *for me* as a food addict. I had already tried different approaches and different food plans in my search for relief. Eventually, I got sick and tired of being sick and tired. *Full of Faith (or full of food?)* is *my* testimony. It is my experience, strength and hope and *my* conclusion thus far. I humbly admit that I only know what I know. I can only share what God has revealed to me in my years of abstinence, and I admit that there are different strokes for different folks.

I strongly encourage everyone to consider a *healthy** plan of eating. With the help of God, it is best to consult with a physician, dietitian or nutritionist for the best solution to an individual's dietary needs. Abstinence (recovery from overeating and food obsession) is having a plan of eating and doing that plan, whatever it is.

The 12-steps from the Christian perspective and the outreach ministry of *Full of Faith* go beyond the physical— beyond the food plan. Emotional and spiritual healing comes with God's Word realized and activated. We can share our love and knowledge of Jesus and let go of the differences in our individual committed food plans.

The Food Addiction Institute (FAI) has produced current scientific evidence that many (if not most) people who struggled with food cravings, found freedom when they eliminated sugar and flour from their plans of eating. In time, other trigger foods are noted and thus eliminated. For me, artificial sweeteners was a necessary culprit that caused cravings. Caffeine, too, had to go for long-term, lasting peace.

> "So whether you eat or drink or whatever you do, do it all for the glory of God." (1 Corinthians 10:31, *New International Version*)

*I believe that a healthy plan of eating should include the basics for good nutrition—a good balance of proteins, grains, vegetables, fruits, dairy and fats.

Why Can't I Stop Overeating?

> "For some people, foods can be as addictive as alcohol," Kay Sheppard tells us. "Gummy bears and marshmallow chicks can be vicious killers whose effects can lead to depression, irritability and even suicide. The terrible truth is that for certain individuals, refined carbohydrates can trigger the addictive process." (Kay Sheppard, *Food Addiction: The Body Knows*, Health Communications, Inc., back cover)

Food Addiction holds unique challenges. *I believe* that a person seeking recovery from overeating and food obsession needs to learn how to nourish a healthy body while at the same time abstaining from addictive foods. To the food addict, sugar and flour cause insurmountable cravings and overeating is inevitable. As the disease progresses, physical and emotional manifestations become increasingly apparent; excess weight, low self-esteem and depression are common symptoms.

The Food Addiction Institute, (www.foodaddictioninstitute.org) documents evidence that a chemical imbalance exists in the physical and psychological make-up of a food addict.

For me, the intricacies of science and medicine are informative, yet pale in comparison to my personal realization that I could not stop overeating for any significant length of time until I stopped eating refined carbohydrates. I tried. God knows I tried. Year after year, I pleaded, "God, heal me. I cannot stop overeating." He ignored my request, so I asked Him again, and again and again. I continued to overeat despite constant attempts to diet and persistent prayer. One day I heard, "God can move mountains; bring your shovel."

On July 23, 1988, I dug in, so to speak. I surrendered my will and my life over to the care of God, and I opened my mind and listened to people who were like me, but had found a way out of their self-destructive behaviors.

For five years, I ate three meals a day with nothing in between except black coffee, black tea and water. Sugar and flour were considered off limits with absolutely no ands, ifs or buts. I stopped overeating and I started walking toward the light.

> "[Jesus said], 'I am the Bread of Life. No one coming to me will ever be hungry again. Those believing in me will never thirst.'" (John 6:35, *The Living Bible*)

As time passed, my plan of eating evolved. I stopped eating wheat, I stopped using caffeine and artificial sweeteners, and I added a metabolic adjustment in the form of a snack to my daily regime.

In 2001, I walked into my doctor's office for my annual physical exam feeling particularly blessed with wellness. We talked about my healthy lifestyle, and I received the usual praises and "job well done" remarks. The exam ended with a trip to the lab for some blood work. From there I was sent to the X-ray Department for my first bone density test to check for osteoporosis. It was routine procedure for women over forty-five.

I wasn't concerned. Through the years, I had listened to the medical professionals and followed their advice. When I stopped menstruating, around the year 1990 due to a thyroid disorder, my doctor prescribed hormone replacement therapy. He told me that I needed to protect myself from osteoporosis. On that same note, my nutritionist set up my food plan to include generous amounts of calcium, and I took a vitamin supplement for my vitamin D and magnesium. In other words, I had done my homework. I was a "good" girl.

A week after my physical exam, I received a phone call from my doctor's office. Stunned by the words coming through the wires, I stuttered, "Osteoporosis? I have the bone mass of an eighty-year old woman, 71% in hip and 68% in my spine? There must be a mistake. I eat three yogurts a day. I take vitamin D with magnesium, even hormone replacement therapy. How can I have osteoporosis?"

My future flashed before me. I would be an old woman perched up with pillows in her wheelchair promoting food addiction recovery. *Why did God ask me to write a book and give me this?* Mystified and angry at traditional medicine, I considered my options.

A natural health care professional answered some of my questions. She explained the theory and importance of balancing proteins, carbohydrates and fats for optimal health. My initial plan of eating included healthy choices, even 1500 mg of calcium daily, but apparently not enough fats to transport the vitamins and minerals throughout my body. This woman told me that Dr. Barry Sears had designed a food plan that might work for me. It was the highly publicized and acclaimed Zone Diet.

Compulsive I bought all the Zone books and prayerfully considered Dr. Sears' research. Even though his work is explained in technical terms for the analytical mind, I did not need to be a rocket scientist to see that the Zone Diet was a workable food plan for me. I continued to respect the disease of food addiction and applied appropriate restrictions, the most prevalent being the avoidance of all sugar and flour products, as it is with any food addict's plan of eating. It wasn't long before I fine-tuned the plan into the "Step Easy Food Plan."

Step Easy Food Plans

> Jesus said, "Come to me, all of you who are weary and carry heavy burdens, and I will give you rest. Take my yoke upon you. Let me teach you, because I am humble and gentle, and you will find rest for your souls. For my yoke fits perfectly, and the burden I give you is light." (Matthew 12:29-30, *New Living Translation*.)

"Step easy" into recovery from overeating and food obsession, clarity of mind, a life of sane and happy usefulness with the help of Jesus. The Step Easy Food Plan incorporates a healthy mix of protein, carbohydrate and fat. My hope is to encourage people to take a step toward wellness with an "Easy does it, but do it" approach.

As with any new food plan, it is best to consult with your physician regarding your individual dietary needs. I disclaim responsibility for any adverse effects arising from the suggestions offered in *Full of Faith (or full of food?)*.

People who are addicted to specific foods and excess foods, like me, need to pay close attention to specifics and the little extras, the things that seem like no big deals, but can make the difference between staying abstinent or succumbing to the disease one more time. For me, in addition to refraining from addictive foods, I weigh and measure my food, and I refrain from extra bites, licks or tastes.

Suggestions for Food Addicts Like Me:

Eliminate all sugar products from your food plan.

Check all food labels for hidden sugar, which can take the form of honey, molasses, brown sugar, corn syrup, barley malt, dextrin, maltodextrin, sorbitol, and most ingredients ending with "ose," including, but not limited to dextrose, sucrose, and maltodextrose.

Eliminate all flour products from your food plan.

Foods in this category include most breads, pastas, all sweets, most cold cereals, the list is extensive, including bagels, doughnuts, muffins and the like. Also, note that flour is often used as a thickening agent in soups, sauces and gravies, and breadcrumbs are used as a binding agent in the preparation of meatloaf or meatballs. *Check labels carefully*.

Limit (or eliminate) caffeine

Best to limit caffeine to no more than 2 cups a day. If caffeine is addictive, wean off caffeine gradually.

Eliminate all alcohol

Some people say that alcohol is liquid sugar with a kick. It is not an option for a food addict.

Limit (or eliminate) artificial sweeteners

Includes all diet drinks and packets of artificial sweeteners added to coffee or tea, plus any artificially sweetened foods.

Use a digital scale and be honest

I find freedom in weighing my food on a digital scale. There is less room for playing games. Honesty is the key. 4 oz. is 4.0 oz—not 4.1 oz. or 4.2 oz. I do use measuring spoons for my fats, although some people prefer to use the scale for everything. 0.5 oz of oil is equal to one tablespoon.

Beverages

Best to drink water (hot or cold) with optional wedge of lemon or lime, seltzer water, herb teas, decaffeinated black coffee or tea.

Never eat standing

It is best to take the time to sit and eat your whole meal at one time, if possible. It is dangerous for a food addict to eat standing at the kitchen counter or to eat piece-meal, even if it is our weighed and measured food. It is much

to take a breather. Sit, relax, and enjoy the meal and the

time. It is a positive self-discipline that gives us an opportunity to say, "I need to replenish my physical, emotional, and spiritual energy." God blesses those decisions.

Pray before each meal

Before I put even one iota of food in my mouth, I pray. I take a moment to say, "Thank You, God, for my abstinence. Thank You for the food on my plate." However, I don't stop there. I am sure to say, "Lord, is this guilt-free?" Then I listen. *I really listen.*

Restaurant dining can be a challenge. Sometimes God tells me that my portions are too big. I then have the opportunity to fix it before I eat my meal. I simply put the excess food on my bread plate and ask again, "Lord, is it guilt-free now?"

This is a simple program, but it's not always easy. As a food addict, I occasionally want to eat foods that are not mine to eat, but with the amazing love and grace of God, I practice my program one day at a time.

Step Three—turning my will and my life over to the care of God, which means I surrender all (even my food) over to His care each day.

The Step Easy Food Plan for Women

Breakfast

6 oz. low-fat milk or plain nonfat yogurt (or 2 or protein exchanges)

1 egg or ½ cup egg substitutes (or l protein exchange)

1 oz. oatmeal, measured dry, cooked with water (or 1 grain/hearty vegetables exchange)
4 oz. fruit (1 fruit exchange)

Optional: ½ tablespoon oil or ½ tablespoon butter (or 1 fat exchange)

Lunch

3 oz. protein (or 3 protein exchanges)

4 oz. potato or 3 oz. rice or 4 oz. kidney beans (or l grain/hearty vegetables exchange)
6-8 oz. salad *and* 6-8 oz. low-carbohydrate vegetables, cooked

1 tablespoon olive oil (or 2 fat exchanges)

Dinner

3 oz. protein (or 3 protein exchanges)

4 oz. potato or 3 oz. rice or 4 oz. kidney beans (or 1 grain/hearty vegetables exchange)

6-8 oz. salad *and* 6-8 oz. low-carbohydrate vegetables, cooked

1 tablespoon olive oil (or 2 fat exchanges)

Metabolic Adjustment*

6 oz. low-fat milk or plain nonfat yogurt (or 2 protein exchanges)

4 oz. fruit (1 fruit exchange)

*If you want a 301 meal plan (3 meals a day with nothing in between), the metabolic adjustment can be added to lunch or dinner.

This is *not* a program of deprivation. There can be some flexibility in setting up a food plan. Depending on age, body size, activity level and metabolism, a person might need more food to sustain their energy level and to avoid physical hunger. I have listed the suggested range in choosing portion sizes.

Breakfast

6-8 oz. low-fat milk or plain nonfat yogurt (or 2 protein exchanges)

1 or 2 eggs (or 1 or 2 protein exchanges)

1 oz. or 1.5 oz whole grain cereal (measured dry) or 4-6 oz. potato (or 1 or 1½ grain/hearty vegetable exchanges)

4-6oz fruit (or 1 or 1 ½ fruit exchanges)

Optional: ½ tablespoon oil or ½ tablespoon butter (or 1 fat exchange)

Lunch:

3 or 4 oz. protein (3 or 4 protein exchanges)

Optional: 4-6 oz. potato or 3-4 oz. rice or 4-6 oz. kidney beans (or 1 or 1½ grain/hearty vegetable exchanges)

6-8 oz. salad *and* 6-8 oz. low-carbohydrate vegetables, cooked

½ or 1 tablespoon olive oil (or 1 or 2 fat exchanges)

Dinner:

3 or 4 oz. protein (3 or 4 proteins exchanges)

4-6 oz. potato or 3-4 oz. rice or 4-6 oz. kidney beans (or 1 or 1½ grain/hearty vegetable exchanges)

6-8 oz. salad *and* 6-8 oz. low-carbohydrate vegetables, cooked

½ or 1 tablespoon olive oil (or 1 or 2 fat exchanges)

Metabolic Adjustment:

6-8 oz. low-fat milk or plain nonfat yogurt (or 2 protein exchanges)

4-6 oz. fruit (1-1½ fruit exchanges)

Step Easy Food Plan for Men

Breakfast:

6-8 oz. low-fat milk or plain nonfat yogurt (or 2 protein exchanges)

2 eggs or ½ cup egg substitute or ½ cup cottage cheese (or 2 protein exchanges)

1.5 oz.–2 oz. whole-grain cereal (measured dry) or 6-8 oz. potatoes (1½ or 2 grain/hearty vegetable exchanges)

6-8 oz fruit (1½-2 fruit exchanges)

Optional: ½-1 tablespoon oil or ½-1 tablespoon butter (or 1 or 2 fat exchanges)

Lunch:

4-6 oz. protein (4 or 6 protein exchanges)

6-8 oz. potato or 4-6 oz. rice or 6-8 oz. kidney beans (or 1½ or 2 grain/hearty vegetable exchanges)

8 oz. salad *and* 8 oz. low-carbohydrate vegetables, cooked

1-1.5 tablespoon olive oil (or 2 or 3 fat exchanges)

Dinner:

4-6 oz. protein (4 or 6 protein exchanges)

6-8 oz. potato or 4-6 oz. rice or 6-8 oz. kidney beans (or 1½ or 2 grain/hearty vegetable exchanges)

8 oz. salad *and* 8 oz. low-carbohydrate vegetables, cooked

1-1.5 tablespoon olive oil (or 2 or 3 fat exchanges)

Metabolic Adjustment:

6-8 oz. low-fat milk or plain nonfat yogurt (or 2 protein exchanges)

6-8 oz fruit (1 ½-2 fruit exchanges)

Remember the definition of abstinence: Plan what you do and do what you plan.

You could use the Step Easy Food Plan as a guideline for a healthy way of eating. Make the decision to have either the minimum or maximum amount for each category (dairy, proteins, grains/starches, fruits, vegetables and fats). Then monitor your weight on a weekly, bi-weekly or monthly basis. You can deduct or add food to your daily regime according to your results.

Food Exchanges—each portion is one exchange

Proteins (exchanges include seafood, poultry, red meats, vegetarian options and dairy):

1 oz. chicken, turkey, 1.5 oz. fish/seafood (tuna, canned in water, haddock, cod, salmon, halibut, bass, catfish,

crabmeat, shrimp, lobster, scallops), 1 oz. beef, pork, lamb, veal, Canadian bacon, 3 strips turkey bacon, 1 egg or ½ cup egg substitute, 2 egg whites, 2 oz. tofu, ½ soy patty, ¼ cup (2 oz.) low-fat cottage cheese, 0.5 oz. hard cheese*

*Hard cheese is high in fat and is best avoided or eaten in very limited amounts.

Prepare proteins by roasting, stewing, grilling, baking or pan-frying in your allotment of olive oil or butter. Deep-fried fish, seafood or chicken is not an option for a food addict.

Grains (exchanges include cereals, hearty vegetables, rice, beans and legumes):

Whole-grain cereals: 1 oz. (measured dry, then cooked with water): Oatmeal, oat bran, grits, Cream of Rice, Cream of Buckwheat, Cream of Barley, Cream of Rye. *Always check cereal labels for sugar, flour, wheat and artificial sweeteners.*

Hearty vegetables (exchanges include rice/beans/legumes): 3 oz. prepared rice (brown preferred) or 4 oz. baked, boiled or mashed potatoes, sweet potatoes, yams, acorn squash, butternut squash, spaghetti squash or cooked green peas, beets, pumpkin, corn (or 1 ear corn on the cob), lentils, chick peas, lima beans, kidney beans, navy beans (or any cooked dried beans)

Avoid French fries or chips of any kind and all wheat and flour products—even "healthy" choices like whole-grain bread and pasta, and note that most gravies, soups and sauces are thickened with flour. Therefore, these foods are considered taboo for a food addict. (Men are allowed 1½-2 servings of grain/hearty vegetables for breakfast, lunch and dinner.)

Low-carbohydrate vegetables (Prepared in a salad, cooked or eaten raw):

Alfalfa sprouts, asparagus, beans (green or wax), Bok choy, broccoli, Brussel sprouts, cabbage, carrots, cauliflower, celery, collard greens, cucumber, eggplant, green or red peppers, kale, lettuce (all varieties), mushrooms, okra, onions, radishes, spinach, Swiss chard, tomatoes, turnips, turnip greens, yellow squash (summer), zucchini, (A 6oz can of V-8 juice or tomato juice can be substituted for a serving of vegetables.)

Fruits (fresh, frozen or canned in its own juice):

4 oz. apple, nectarine, orange, peach, pear, plum, tangerine, applesauce, apricots, blackberries, blueberries, cantaloupe,

½grapefruit, 4 oz. grapes,* honeydew melon, pineapple,* raspberries, strawberries, watermelon, 4 oz. canned fruit in its own juice

*Grapes and pineapple have been known to set up cravings in some food addicts. Consider your options carefully and listen to your body when introducing these foods.

Note of caution when considering bananas and dried fruits: Bananas are high in sugar. It is best to avoid them; however, if a banana is "doctor recommended," the portion size is 1/2 banana or 2.5 oz.

Dried fruits are also high in sugar. Therefore they are not generally considered "safe" foods; however if prunes need to be incorporated into your plan of eating for health reasons, treat them like a prescription drug. Pray that God will protect you from the potentially harmful excess of natural sugar in this food choice.

Fats (1 fat exchange contains approximately 5-7 grams of fat):1 tablespoon regular *sugar-free* salad dressing, ½ tablespoon olive oil, ½ tablespoon canola oil, ½ tablespoon sesame oil, ½ tablespoon butter, ½ tablespoon real mayonnaise, ½ tablespoon coconut oil, ½ tablespoon flax oil

Condiments:

2 tablespoons mustard, 2 tablespoons sugar-free salsa per meal, vinegar

Ground flax seeds are considered a healthy supplement—up to 3 tablespoons daily

Beverages:

Wonderful, life-giving water (hot or cold) with optional wedge of lemon or lime, seltzer water, herb teas, decaffeinated *black* coffee and tea

Five Sample Days—Step Easy Food Plan for Women:

Day One:

Breakfast: 6 oz. plain nonfat yogurt, l egg, l oz. oatmeal, 4 oz. peach, (optional: ½ tablespoon olive oil)

Lunch: 3 oz. chicken, 4 oz. baked potato, 8 oz. broccoli, 8 oz. salad, 1 tablespoon olive oil

Dinner: 4 oz. haddock, 3 oz. brown rice, 8 oz. green beans, 8 oz. salad, 2 tablespoon Newman's Own Olive Oil and Vinegar Salad Dressing

Metabolic: ½ cup cottage cheese, 4 oz. unsweetened applesauce

Day Two:

Breakfast: 6 oz. low-fat milk, 2 oz. cottage cheese, l oz. oat bran, 4 oz. apple, (optional: ½ tablespoon flax oil)

Lunch: 3 oz. turkey, 4 oz. kidney beans, 8 oz. cauliflower, 8 oz. salad, 2 tablespoon Newman's Own Olive Oil and Vinegar Salad Dressing

Dinner: 3 oz. ground beef with 2 tablespoons sugar-free salsa, 4 oz. boiled potatoes, 8 oz. broccoli, 8 oz salad, 1 tablespoon olive oil

Metabolic: 2 oz. chicken, 4 oz. plum

Day Three:

Breakfast: 6 oz. low-fat milk, ½ cup egg substitute, 1 oz. Cream of Rye, 4 oz. crushed pineapple, (optional: ½ tablespoon olive oil)

Lunch: 4 oz. salmon, 3 oz. brown rice, 8 oz. broccoli and cauliflower, 8 oz. salad, 1 tablespoon olive oil

Dinner: 3 oz. pork, 4 oz. baked potato, 8 oz. summer squash, 8 oz. salad, 1 tablespoon butter

Metabolic: 6 oz. plain nonfat yogurt, 4 oz. blueberries.

Day Four:

Breakfast: 6 oz. low-fat milk, 1 egg, 1 oz. oat bran, 4 oz. orange, (optional: ½ tablespoon olive oil)

Lunch: 6 oz. cottage cheese, 4 oz. kidney beans, 16 oz. salad, 2 tablespoon Newman's Own Olive Oil and Vinegar Salad Dressing

Dinner: 3 oz. steak, 3 oz brown rice, 8 oz. turnip, 8 oz. salad, 1 tablespoon olive oil

Metabolic: 6 oz. skim milk, 4 oz. apple

Day Five:

Breakfast: 2 eggs (in place of the dairy), 0.5 oz cheddar cheese, 4 oz. potatoes, 4 oz. strawberries, (optional: ½ tablespoon butter)

Lunch: 3 oz. ground beef, 2 tablespoons sugar-free salsa, 4 oz. baked potato, 8 oz. cauliflower, 8 oz salad, 1 tablespoon olive oil

Dinner: 3 oz. chicken, 3 oz. brown rice, 16 oz onions, peppers, mushrooms, tomatoes, broccoli (stir-fried in 1 tablespoon olive oil)

Metabolic: 6 oz. plain nonfat yogurt, 4 oz. nectarine

Live and Let Live

Eating at a restaurant can be challenging because there are so many temptations. However, with a determined mindset and dependence on God's help, it is possible to stay on the Step Easy Food Plan. Some recovering food addicts bring a digital scale and measuring spoons to any dining experience, while others prefer to practice the eyeball method. In either case, recovering food addicts do not indulge in excessive quantities, and they do not forfeit the sugar, flour, wheat, artificial sweeteners boundary.

For *breakfast,* you could have an egg, oatmeal or grits, a glass of milk and a fresh fruit or a small glass of juice, although juice is not usually a recommended choice. Another option is two eggs or a vegetable omelet, home fries and a piece of fruit. Occasionally, I order one or two eggs,

Canadian bacon, home fries and maybe a piece of fruit. It is not the usual plan, but we need to remember the definition of abstinence: "Plan what you do and do what you plan."

For *lunch or dinne*r, you could order broiled or grilled chicken, fish or beef with a baked potato or rice. Bring your digital scale or cut the protein to the size of a deck of cards and cut the potato in half. If rice is your choice and you choose not to weigh or measure it, eyeball it to equal 1/2 cup. Order a salad and a cooked vegetable if they are available without added sugar or sauce. Note that coleslaw, butternut squash and carrots are often laced with sugar. It is best to use oil and vinegar for a garden or Caesar salad or bring your salad dressing in a small container from home. I strongly suggest avoiding restaurant salad dressing unless you are certain that it is sugar-free.

Another option is a grilled chicken Caesar salad. Order it without the croutons or the salad dressing. Use your own dressing or oil and vinegar. If it is an option, order a baked potato and cut it in half or order another hearty vegetable like corn on the cob to make the meal complete. Sometimes I order a glass of tomato juice as a supplement to my low-carbohydrate vegetable allotment.

At a *salad bar* choose plain vegetables such as lettuce, onions, tomatoes, cucumbers, mushrooms, green peppers, radishes, broccoli and the like, without sauces or marinates of any kind. Sugar or excess fat lurks in choices like three-bean salad, coleslaw or marinated mushrooms.

Chinese restaurants offer suitable meals. A common lunch or dinner for a food addict consists of steamed or stir-fried vegetables with chicken, shrimp or beef and white or brown rice. Some people measure the rice in the Chinese teacup. It might not be exact, but it is a boundary. Note that fried rice has added sugar. As an added precaution, I always say "no sugar please" when ordering anything at a Chinese restaurant.

In recent years, many *fast-food restaurants* have added healthier choices to their menus. If you need a quick meal and you cannot find a restaurant that offers a salad/protein combination, you could order a plain salad and a hamburger or grilled chicken sandwich. Throw away the roll. Use oil and vinegar or bring your salad dressing from home. Order a baked potato and eat half to make the meal complete or have a fruit* instead of the potato.

*I usually bring emergency food with me when I leave my home or I stop at a market to buy whatever I need if I find myself in a pinch.

Whether you are at home or on the road, it is important to pay attention to your feelings. In other words, *halt* before you overeat or make poor choices. Don't get too hungry, angry, lonely or tired.

On the days when I am *physically ill*, I continue to follow my plan of eating to the best of my ability. It is okay to substitute a breakfast-type meal for lunch or dinner; I often have scrambled eggs and oatmeal with unsweetened applesauce when I am "under the weather." Sometimes I make chicken soup by simmering chicken on the stove. I measure 3 oz. of chicken, 3 oz. or rice and 6 oz. cooked carrots. I add a cup or two of the broth after skimming the excess fat, which floats to the top when the broth is cooled. If I am too sick to eat all my food for the day, I let it go and pray for health and acceptance of life on life's terms.

Note: If I need medications, I always check the labels for sugar. Sometimes I need to ask the pharmacist to suggest sugar-free alternatives.

Step Easy Maintenance Food Plan

When you reach your goal weight, it is time to consider adding more food to your daily plan of eating. Introduce foods gradually. As a first step, you could double the fat portions at lunch and dinner. If your weight does not stabilize, then increase the protein at lunch and dinner. After that, increase the size of your fruits or add another fruit to lunch or dinner.

Ups and Downs

On my way down the scale, I hit times when the scale didn't budge. It was downright discouraging, but I soon learned that the usual culprits for me were too many high-fat protein choices and/or too frequent restaurant dining experiences. In order to get back into lose-weight mode, I simply went back to basics. I stayed home and ate low-fat protein until the scale started moving again.

That worked for many years until I grew older and my metabolism changed. At that point, in order to stay at goal weight, I eliminated the serving of grain/hearty vegetable at lunch and dinner. With that simple reduction, I continued to stay at my maintenance weight. It was not hard. Therefore, I assumed that my body didn't need the extra food I had been eating.

This is an example my revised maintenance plan in 2004, which could be lose-weight mode for an overweight woman.

Breakfast:

6 oz. plain nonfat yogurt

1 egg or ½ cup egg substitutes

1 oz. oatmeal (measured dry) (or another whole-grain cereal)

½ tablespoon butter or coconut oil

2 tablespoon ground flax seeds

Lunch:

3 oz. protein

8 oz. salad and 8 oz. low-carbohydrate vegetables, cooked

1 tablespoon olive oil

Dinner:

3 oz. protein

8 oz. salad and low-carbohydrate vegetables, cooked

1 grain/starch exchange*

1 tablespoon olive oil

Before bed:

6 oz. plain nonfat yogurt

1 small/medium sized fruit

½ tablespoon butter or coconut oil

1 tablespoon ground flax seeds

*Or I have 1 oz. of Oatmeal or Oat bran with my last meal of the day.

This plan worked for me. I am smiling because I have said that many times through the years. Each step in my one-day-at-a-time life worked until God told me to do something different.

Farewell—Follow the Cloud

This is *a rich and rewarding new way of life*. When you make the decision to follow a committed plan of eating, it is possible to stay abstinent and free from compulsive overeating and food obsession. Your new mindset will replace the old self-destructive tapes that once controlled your life. Start with words like "I think I can. I think I can. I think I can."

> Jesus told them, "I assure you, even if you had faith as small as a mustard seed, you could say to this mountain, 'Move from here to there,' and it

would move. Nothing would be impossible."
(Matthew 17:20, *New Living Translation*)

God wants us to be happy and He wants us to succeed. The momentum will flow. Do your 1%, which is following a food plan, and God will carry you from there. Soon you will be saying, "Thank you, Jesus, for another day of abstinence." If you can find the willingness to join me in recovery, you will find a peace and clarity that passes all understanding.

> "Trust in the Lord and do good. Then you will live safely in the land and prosper. Take delight in the Lord, and he will give you your heart's desire. Commit everything you do to the Lord. Trust Him, and he will help you. (Psalm 37:3-5, *New Living Translation*)

God bless you as you consider this difficult, yet life-changing challenge. Visit our web site: www.fulloffaith.com and join one of our blogs for personal interaction, support and encouragement. You would be welcomed.

> God is faithful. "...God, who began the good work within you, will continue his work until it is finally finished..." (Philippians 1:6, *New Living Translation*)

Bibliography
Alcoholics Anonymous, third edition, New York: Alcoholics Anonymous World Service, 1976.

Friends in Recovery, *The Twelve Steps for Christians,* Revised Edition, California: RPI Publishing, Inc., 1994.

Sears, Barry, *A Week in the Zone,* New York, HarperCollins, 2000.

Sears, Barry, *Mastering The Zone,* New York, HarperCollins, 1997.

Sheppard, Kay, *Food Addiction: The Body Knows,* Revised Edition, Florida: Health Communications, Inc., l993.

The Amplified Bible, Michigan: Zondervan Corporation and California: The Lockman Foundation, 1987.

The Holy Bible, New International Version, Michigan: Zondervan Publishing House and International Bible Society, l984.

The Holy Bible, The New Living Translation, Illinois: Tyndale House Publishers, Inc., l996.

The Living Bible, Illinois: Tyndale House Publishers, Inc., 1971.

agrees with the views expressed herein. A.A. is a program of recovery from alcoholism <u>only</u> – use of the Twelve Steps in connection with programs and activities which are patterned after A.A., but which address other problems, or in any other non-A.A. context, does not imply otherwise. Additionally, while A.A. is a spiritual program, A.A. is not a religious program. Thus, A.A. is not affiliated or allied with any sect, denomination, or specific religious belief.

Statement of Faith
I believe in...

...**One God,** the Father, Son and Holy Spirit, who created all things by His almighty power and is in control of all things.

...**The Bible**, which is God's Word, and tells us all we need to know about what we should believe and how we should live.

...**Man**, who was created perfect in the image of God, but who through disobedience became a slave of sin and liable to God's justice.

...**Jesus Christ**, the eternal Son of God, who became man, lived a sinless life and died in our place, taking away our guilt; who rose physically from the dead and is alive and reigning in heaven today as Lord of all; who will one day come again to this world and judge all people, condemning those who are impenitent and unbelieving, and taking to glory with Him those who have truly believed in Him.

...**The Holy Spirit**, who works in the hearts of sinners, enabling them to believe in Jesus Christ and to repent of their sins, and who is a living reality in the lives of those who are true believers.

...**The Forgiveness of Sin**, which comes about as God's free and undeserved gift through the death of Jesus Christ and is received only through faith in Him.

...**The Church,** which is the world-wide community of all who truly believe in the Lord Jesus Christ.

Scripture Index:

Introduction
Matthew 5:6 (NIV)

Reach for a Star
Matthew 17:21-22 (NLT)

Chapter One: Realization
Psalm 119:25 (NLT)

Chapter Two: Acceptance
Isaiah 61:4 (NIV)

Twinkle, Twinkle Little Star
(Refers to Romans 5:1, John 3:16, Romans 3:23, 6:23, Proverbs 14:12, Isaiah 59:2, 1 Timothy 2:5, 1 Peter 3:18a, Revelations 3:20, John 1:12, Romans 10:9, Romans 10:13, Ephesians 2:8-9)

Jack and Jill Went Up the Hill
Mark 9:23-24 (LIV)

Chapter Three: Surrender
Psalm 40:2 (NLT)

Follow the Yellow Brick Road
Matthew 11:28 (NIV)

Chapter Four: Action
Proverbs 3:5-6 (NIV)

Ruffled Feathers
1 Peter 5:7-9 (NLT)

The Real Deal
Proverbs 3:5-6 (NIV)

One Day at a Time
Philippians 4:11 (AMP), Psalm 46:1 (NIV), Lamentations 3:21-23 (NIV)

I Think I Can...My First Baking Experience
Ecclesiastes 4:9-12 (NLT)

I Think I Can...My First Wedding Reception
Matthew 6:34 (NLT)

Touchdown
1 Timothy 4:8 (NLT)

New Light
Isaiah 61:1-7 (NLT), Matthew 5:6 (NIV) Psalm 119:18-20 (LIV)

Higher Ground
1 Corinthians 13:11 (NIV), Proverbs 12:15 (NLT)

A Leap of Faith
Psalm 32:8 (NIV), Isaiah 40:31 (NIV), 1 Corinthians 13:4-8 (NIV)

There's No Place Like Home
Matthew 18:20 (NIV)

Rise and Shine
2 Peter 1:5-8 (NIV), Romans 12:6-8 (NIV), (refers to Philippians 1:6)

Good to the Last Drop
Romans 12:1-2 (NLT), 1 Corinthians 10:23 (NIV), John 8:36 (NLT)

The Good Fight
2 Chronicles 20:12 (NLT), 2 Chronicles 20:15-17 (NLT), Philippians 3:13-14 (NLT)

Living Free
Philippians 4:11-13 (NIV), Jeremiah 29:11 (NLT)

An Attitude of Gratitude
Romans 12:2 (NLT), Psalm 46:1 (NLT), Philippians 4:4-7 (NLT), refers to Lamentations 3:23, Philippians 4:l9, Romans l4:l7

A Heart for God
Hebrews 12:2 (NIV), Psalm 37:3-5 (NLT), Ephesians 2:lo (NLT)

Dare to Dream
Ephesians 3:20 (NLT), Ephesians 3:17-21 (NLT)

Chapter Five—Recovery
Isaiah 30:21 (NIV), Isaiah 61:2-3 (LIV)

It's Electric
Hebrews 11:1 (LIV), John 8:12 (LIV), John 14:27 (AMP)

The Serenity Prayer with Scripture
2 Timothy 4:16-17, (NLT), Philippians 4:6-7 (NLT), Philippians 4:11 (AMP), Psalm 37:5 (LIV), Proverbs 3:5-6 (AMP), Lamentations 3:22-23 (RSV), Psalm 118:24 (NIV), Psalm 46:l (NIV), 2 Corinthians 4:8-10 (NLT), Romans 8:28 (NLT), Psalm 28:7 (NLT), Psalm 23:6 (NIV), John 3:16 (AMP)

Heart to Heart—Are You a Food Addict Like Me?
John 8:32 (NLT), Romans 7:18 (NLT)

You've Got a Friend
Ecclesiastes 4:9-10, 12 (NIV)

Slow and Steady Wins the Race
1 Corinthians 10:23 (NIV), Romans 14:17 (NLT), (refers to Romans 7-7, Ephesians 2:8-9, Luke 18:17, Genesis 3,

Galatians 5:23), Matthew 7:7 (NIV), John 14:16 (AMP), Matthew 6:6-8 (NLT), Ecclesiastes 4:9-10, 12 (NIV), Matthew 18:20 (NIV), Psalm 119:18-20 (LIV), (refers to Matthew 5:13-16), Matthew 7:12 (NLT), Romans 12:9-10, 16 (LIV)

The Elevator is Broken—Try the Steps
Romans 12:1-2 (NLT), Matthew 5:8 (AMP)

The Twelve Steps and Relevant Scripture
Psalm 119:25 (LIV), Psalm 119:18-20 (LIV), Proverbs 3:5-6 (NIV), Galatians 6:4 (AMP), James 5:16 (AMP), Proverbs 3:11-12 (LIV), 1 John 1:9 (LIV), Luke 6:31 (NIV), Colossians 3:13 (NIV), Ephesians 4:23-25 (LIV), Ephesians 6:18 (NLT), 2 Corinthians 4:1 (LIV)

Chapter Six—Food Plans/Abstinence
1 Corinthians 10:23 (NIV)

Different Strokes for Different Folks
Galatians 5:22-23 (LIV), 1 Corinthians 10:31 (NIV)

Why Can't I Stop Overeating?
John 6:35 (LIV)

Step Easy Food Plan
Matthew 12:29-30 (NLT)

Live and Let Live
Matthew 17:20 (NLT), Psalm 37:3-5 (NLT)

The Twelve Steps of Alcoholics Anonymous®

Step one: We admitted we were powerless over alcohol—that our lives had become unmanageable.

Step two: Came to believe that a Power greater than ourselves could restore us to sanity.

Step three: Made a decision to turn our will and our lives over to the care of God as we understood Him.

Step four: Made a searching and fearless moral inventory of ourselves.

Step five: Admitted to God, to ourselves, and to another human being the exact nature of our wrongs.

Step six: Were entirely ready to have God remove all these defects of character.

Step seven: Humbly asked Him to remove our shortcomings.

Step eight: Made a list of all persons we had harmed, and became willing to make amends to them all.

Step nine: Make direct amends to such people wherever possible, except when to do so would injure them or others.

Step ten: Continued to take personal inventory and when we were wrong promptly admitted it.

Step eleven: Sought through prayer and meditation to improve our conscious contact with God as we understood Him, praying only for knowledge of His will for us and the power to carry that out.

Step twelve: Having had a spiritual awakening as the result of these Steps, we tried to carry this message to alcoholics, and to practice these principles in all our affairs.

Alcoholics Anonymous World Services, Inc®

Mission Statement:

Full of Faith, Christian 12-Step Recovery from Food Addiction, exists to touch the heart and minds of the person who struggles (or has struggled) with compulsive or addictive eating. With a disciplined way of eating and lifestyle changes based on Biblical truths, God's love and grace brings transformation and restoration.

Vision:

Testimonies will proclaim Full of Faith as the catalyst to share the good news that Jesus and a Biblical approach to freedom from compulsive and addictive eating brings freedom to those struggling. There will be meetings available by phone and in person around the world. People will get set free. News will spread and more will be set free.

About the author:

Pam Masshardt, author of Sweet Surrender*, Christian 12-step Recovery from Food Addiction, started her ministry, Full of Faith, in the year 2000. On July 23, 2013, she celebrated 25 years of freedom from compulsive overeating. She abstains from sugar, flour, trigger foods, plus amounts. Her book and the website, fulloffaith.com, reveal the intimate details of her testimony.

In 2013, Karen Schoenmaker, a Christian in recovery from food addiction, joined Pam as a faithful contributor, encourager and shepherd. As a writer, communication specialist and educator, Karen walks alongside Pam in the ministry. They advocate for the education and awareness of food addiction, a physical, emotional and spiritual malady for the compulsive and addictive eater. foodaddictioninstition.org verifies evidence that supports their claims.

Sweet Surrender:

Sweet Surrender is an outreach from Full of Faith. It's a weekly phone meeting offering Christian 12-step support and encouragement for the person struggling (or who has struggled) with compulsive or addictive eating. All are welcomed--Christians or people who are not sure about their relationship with God. We use the Bible, The Big Book of Alcoholics Anonymous and the 12-steps to encourage life-style change. Leaders have 90days or more of abstinence, have accountability and have faith in Jesus. They share their personal experience, strength and hope in experiencing a sweet surrender. There are no dues or fees for membership. Sweet Surrender is not a medical group, but follow the guidelines of foodaddictioninstitute.org. For professional help, the group suggests that people refer to http://foodaddiction.com/wp-content/uploads/acorn_brochure.pd

In between meetings, fulloffaith.com offers an interactive blog for questions and comments, plus another blog for accountability, a place where people can commit their specific food plan for the day.

In regards to food plans, we believe that there are different strokes for different folks. However, for those who are looking for a specific food plan that supports the withdrawal process and clean abstinence, we offer an option called "Step Easy". It is a healthy way of eating, no sugar, flour, trigger foods. It is available on the website.

NOTES

NOTES

NOTES

Made in the USA
Lexington, KY
24 July 2014